BEAT CANCER
KITCHEN

Also by Chris Wark

Chris Beat Cancer

Beat Cancer Daily

All of the above are available at your local bookstore, or may be ordered by visiting:

Hay House USA: www.hayhouse.com®
Hay House Australia: www.hayhouse.com.au
Hay House UK: www.hayhouse.co.uk
Hay House India: www.hayhouse.co.in

Published in the United States by: Hay House, Inc.: www.hayhouse.com®
Published in Australia by: Hay House Australia Pty. Ltd.: www.hayhouse.com.au
Published in the United Kingdom by: Hay House UK, Ltd.: www.hayhouse.co.uk
Published in India by: Hay House Publishers India: www.hayhouse.co.in

Indexer: J S Editorial, LLC
Cover design: Shubhani Sarkar
Interior design: Julie Davison
Interior photos: Justin Fox Burks

Library of Congress has cataloged the earlier edition as follows:

Names: Wark, Chris, author. | Wark, Micah, author.
Title: Beat cancer kitchen : deliciously simple plant-based anticancer
    recipes / Chris and Micah Wark.
Description: 1st edition. | Carlsbad, California : Hay House, Inc., [2021]
Identifiers: LCCN 2021032882 | ISBN 9781401961961 (hardback) | ISBN
    9781401961978 (ebook)
Subjects: LCSH: Cancer--Diet therapy--Recipes. | LCGFT: Cookbooks.
Classification: LCC RC271.D52 W37 2021 | DDC 641.5/631--dc23
LC record available at https://lccn.loc.gov/2021032882

Tradepaper ISBN: 978-1-4019-6521-1
E-book ISBN: 978-1-4019-6197-8

10 9 8 7 6 5
1st edition, November 2021
2nd edition, May 2023

Printed in China

BEAT CANCER KITCHEN

KITCHEN

Deliciously Simple Plant-Based Anticancer Recipes

CHRIS & MICAH WARK

Photography by Justin Fox Burks

HAY HOUSE, INC.
Carlsbad, California • New York City
London • Sydney • New Delhi

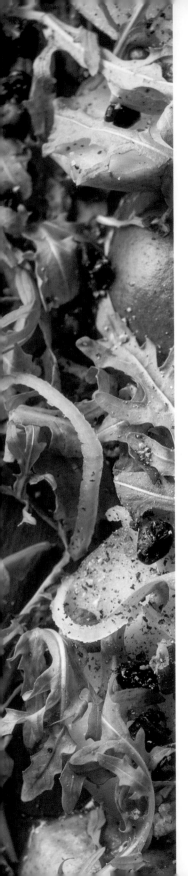

CONTENTS

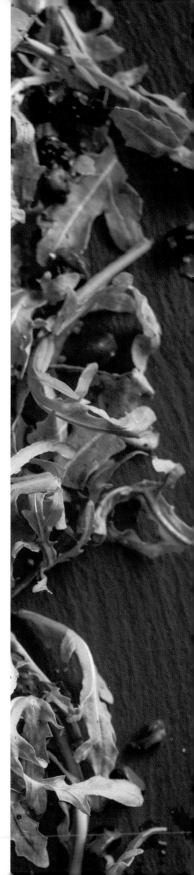

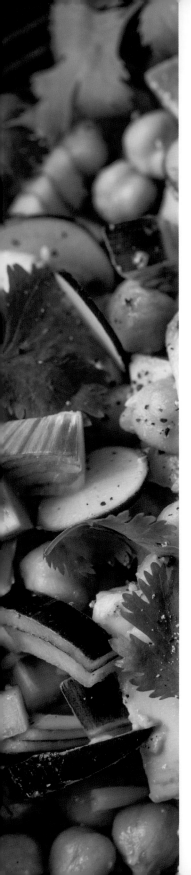

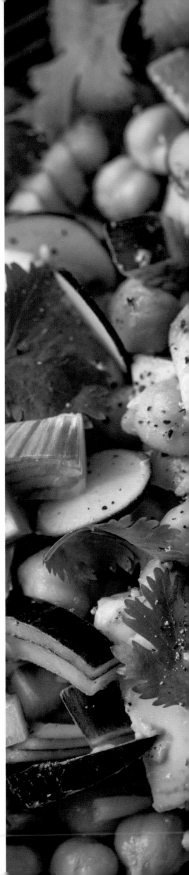

INTRODUCTION

First confession: I'm a terrible cook! I don't have the time or patience for complicated recipes, and I've never been interested in experimenting in the kitchen. I'm a creature of habit. Once I find a meal I like that's super healthy and tastes good, I am perfectly content eating it every day. And for breakfast and lunch that's pretty much what I do. Micah, on the other hand, is a terrific cook. She has come up with some fantastic recipes over the years, and she makes dinner every night for the family. And then I do the dishes (super-husband pro tip).

Second confession: I didn't want to write a cookbook. Writing a cookbook has never been a dream or a goal. It wasn't in my life plan. But hey, neither was cancer . . . and here we are! This book of recipes exists because my incredible community of survivors and thrivers wouldn't leave me alone about it. This book is all your fault. You forced us to take on this project—to get creative and innovate. And now *Beat Cancer Kitchen* is here! Thank you for the encouragement. We are so excited to share our favorite recipes with you.

We lovingly created this book of recipes with the help of a dear friend, who chose to remain anonymous, to show you how easy, delicious, nutritious, adventurous, and fun whole-food plant-based eating can be.

If you haven't yet, I want to encourage you to read my first book, *Chris Beat Cancer: A Comprehensive Plan for Healing Naturally*. In that book I tell my survival story, address the limitations of conventional medicine, and take a deep dive into lifestyle medicine to show you the evidence-based healing power of a whole-food plant-based diet, exercise, stress reduction, a positive mindset, faith, and forgiveness, all of which are not only key to my survival but are common threads connecting many holistic and against-the-odds survivors.

I think it's important to remove the stigma around the word *diet*. We are all on a diet. And your diet is the sum total of the things you choose to eat, especially what you eat the most. The Western diet—the way most people eat in industrialized countries—is a recipe for disease. It is a diet high in animal protein, fat, processed oils, refined grains, sugar, salt, and food additives and low in antioxidants, prebiotic fiber, and thousands of anticancer phytonutrients found only in plant food.

Eating the right food can help your body heal and help prevent chronic illnesses like cardiovascular disease, type 2 diabetes, and many types of cancer. There are powerful compounds in plant food that help to kill cancer cells, block tumor growth, stop the spread of cancer, strengthen your immune system, reduce inflammation, increase detoxification, and prevent healthy cells from ever becoming cancerous in the first place. You want these compounds circulating in your body every day.

You don't need a medical background or a scientific degree or even a high school diploma to understand the simple truth that unprocessed food from the earth is good for you. And the more you eat, the better.

A whole-food plant-based diet rich in fruits, vegetables, legumes, nuts, seeds, whole grains, herbs, and spices is not a crash diet or a fad diet. It is a diet for optimal health and longevity. And the ideal amount of plant food is at least 10 servings per day. I know what you're thinking, *10 servings*? It sounds like a lot, but it really isn't. This is totally doable. One serving is just a cup of raw fruit or vegetables, or half a cup of cooked veggies. A big bowl or plate full of veggies is three to four servings. But there's no need to measure or obsess about how many servings you're getting. For example, if you have oatmeal with flaxseed, blueberries, and walnuts for breakfast, a giant salad for lunch, and a delicious assortment of cooked veggies for dinner, that easily puts you over 10 servings for the day. Snacking on fresh fruit like an apple or on a handful of almonds bumps you up even more. See how easy that is?

Fresh vegetable juice is medicinal food and is supplemental to a healthy diet. Drinking vegetable juice with or between meals will bump you up to 15 to 20 servings of plant food per day. If you are in healing mode, this is what I suggest in order to maximize your anticancer nutrition intake each day. I call this strategy *overdosing on nutrition*.

In my second book, a devotional called *Beat Cancer Daily*, one of the major themes is the power of your daily choices. Your choices each day are creating your future. All of the small changes and small improvements you make to your daily routine add up to massive change over time. That's how nutrition works and how healing happens. No one gets chronic disease overnight, so don't expect to reverse it overnight. But day by day as you continue to take care of yourself in a way that you never have before, you supply your body with an abundance of life-giving nutrients that it will use to repair, regenerate, detoxify, and heal.

Healthy eating isn't hard. It's just a matter of swapping out your usual fare with fresh new dishes that delight, nourish, and satisfy you.

This book is divided into two major sections. The first section is the hard-core anticancer diet, which outlines the simple daily dietary routine that I followed during the most intensive season, the first few years, of my cancer-healing journey. The second section, which makes up the bulk of the recipes, is focused on eating for prevention. It's how we eat now. You will also find fun and fascinating scientific factoids about the anticancer action of specific foods sprinkled throughout this book.

Every recipe in *Beat Cancer Kitchen* is plant-based and lower in salt and oil than what you'll find in traditional cookbooks. Sweeteners include fruit, maple syrup, blackstrap molasses, and honey. Fresh fruits—especially berries—are a delicious source of vitamins, minerals, fiber, probiotics, enzymes, antioxidants, and anticancer nutrients. Don't be afraid of the sugars in fruit. Fruit is not the cause of obesity, chronic disease, or cancer. You don't get cancer from eating too much fruit.

Maple syrup contains antioxidants and anticancer polyphenols such as quebecol and ginnalins, which have been found to inhibit the growth of several types of cancer cells.[1] The darker the syrup, the better.

Blackstrap molasses is the highest-antioxidant sweetener known.[2] It's a great source of iron, calcium, magnesium, and potassium and it has high concentrations of linoleic acid, a known anticancer compound.[3]

For non-vegans, honey is an approved sweetener with unique antimicrobial, immune-supporting, and anticancer properties,[4] and can be substituted one to one for maple syrup, depending on the flavor you are going for. I suggest sourcing honey locally. Farmers' markets are a good place to start, and if you ask around you may find several beekeepers in your circle of friends and family. I happen to know three. One beekeeper works at our kids' school. One works out at my gym, and another one, "Mr. Bill," lives across the street from us. Beekeepers are everywhere!

Finally, in order to not have to type the word *organic* in front of every ingredient in this book, here is our position on organic food. We recommend you use organic ingredients as much as possible. Choosing organic produce reduces your exposure to toxic chemical herbicides, fungicides, and pesticides like atrazine and chlorpyrifos, as well as Roundup, which is a glyphosate-based herbicide that is sprayed on genetically modified crops as well as many conventionally grown crops to dry them out before harvest. A study worth mentioning found that urinary pesticide levels in humans dropped by 89 percent after just one week on an all-organic diet.[5] Pesticides tend to concentrate in the skin of produce. So if you eat the skin, as in apples, celery, kale, or berries, it's more important to buy organic. If you don't eat the skin, as in citrus fruit, melons, or avocados, conventional is okay. If organic produce is not available to you, eat tons of fruits and vegetables anyway. They are still incredible health-supporting foods and the benefits outweigh the risks.

The most effective way to reduce up to 74 percent of pesticides from produce appears to be soaking them in a simple homemade solution of one part salt in nine parts water for 20 minutes.[6]

Fruits, vegetables, mushrooms, nuts, seeds, legumes, whole grains, herbs, and spices are the foundational ingredients of the anticancer diet. The truth is simple: Whole foods from the earth give your body vital nutrients that support healing. The food on the end of your fork has the power to promote health or promote disease. And the intention of this book is to make the whole-food plant-based anticancer diet easy and fun. Welcome to *Beat Cancer Kitchen*!

Love,
Chris and Micah

P.S. ChrisBeatCancer.com is a free online resource with hundreds of articles on prevention and healing as well as interviews with integrative doctors, nutritional science experts, and holistic survivors. If you are looking for inspiration, encouragement, direction, and hope, you will find it there. Join my free email newsletter and dig in!

WHEN TO EAT, WHEN NOT TO EAT

I want to encourage you to eat all of your meals in an 11-hour window each day. This gives you 13 hours of nightly fasting. Late-night eating is a destructive habit that interferes with the incredible healing benefits of sleep and promotes excess body-fat retention and weight gain. As a general rule, it's best to go to bed on an empty stomach several hours after dinner.

For example, if you eat breakfast at 8 A.M., finish dinner by 7 P.M. and aim for a bedtime between 9 and 10 P.M. If you eat breakfast earlier than 8 A.M., have an earlier dinner. Do not skip breakfast and eat only lunch and dinner. Your body processes food most efficiently and burns more calories from food eaten early in the day. One study found that a meal eaten at 8 P.M. caused twice the blood sugar spike in humans as the exact same meal eaten at 8 A.M.[7] A late dinner is like eating double the calories. As the saying goes, eat like a king for breakfast, a prince for lunch, and a pauper for dinner. If you want to lose or maintain weight, breakfast and lunch should be your largest meals. However, if you need to gain weight, eat less for breakfast and more for dinner. Just make sure it's an early dinner.

This simple practice of time-restricted eating has been found to increase weight loss while reducing blood pressure, inflammation, insulin resistance, blood sugar, and oxidative stress. You may also find that you have more energy during the day and sleep better at night.

A study found that breast cancer patients who did not eat their meals within an 11-hour window each day were found to have a 36 percent higher risk of recurrence than those who did.[8] Eating your meals in a smaller 8-hour window with up to 16 hours of nightly fasting could be even more beneficial, especially if you have weight you want to lose.

THE ANIMAL PROTEIN CANCER CONNECTION

The dietary advice given to most cancer patients is at best painfully ignorant and at worst potentially deadly. Cancer patients are routinely told by their doctors and nutritionists to eat whatever they want and are often sent home with suggestions to consume high-calorie junk food like ice cream and milkshakes. In addition, there are a number of cancer diet books with meat-based recipes despite the countless published studies demonstrating how eating animal products can cause and promote cancer growth. Here's why a diet high in animal food is not a good idea for cancer healing and prevention.

In 2015, after reviewing 800 scientific studies, the International Agency for Research on Cancer (IARC) classified processed meats including bacon, sausage, ham, hot dogs, deli meats, canned meat, and jerky as Group 1 carcinogens.[9,10] That means there is sufficient evidence that these foods directly cause cancer. Eating just 1.75 ounces of processed meat per day—that's about two strips of bacon—increases your risk of colorectal cancer by 18 percent.[11] Red meat (beef, pork, lamb, etc.) is classified as a Group 2A carcinogen, which means the current body of evidence indicates that it is a probable cause of cancer. A separate meta-analysis associated consumption of red meat and processed meat with an increased risk of colorectal, esophageal, liver, lung, and pancreatic cancers.[12]

Another notable study found that middle-aged Americans who reported eating a high-protein diet with more than 20 percent of calories coming from animal protein were four times more likely to die of cancer or diabetes, and twice as likely to die of any other cause over the next 18 years. But those who ate a plant-based diet did not have any increase in risk.[13] Aside from processed meat and red meat being potential direct cancer causers, here are six components of animal food that contribute to cancer growth.

Saturated Fat

A diet high in animal protein—meat, dairy, eggs—is also high in saturated fat. A diet high in saturated fat has been found to increase your risk of lung cancer and intestinal cancers.[14,15] A diet high in saturated fat also increases a man's risk of aggressive prostate cancer[16] and a woman's risk of post-menopausal breast cancer[17] and breast cancer death.[18] There is no association of increased cancer risk from saturated fat found in whole plant food such as nuts, seeds, and avocados.

Cholesterol

Dietary cholesterol has been associated with an increased risk of many cancers, including stomach, colorectal, breast, lung, pancreatic, kidney, bladder, and non-Hodgkin's lymphoma.[19] Cholesterol

metabolites support cancer progression and suppress immune responses. Studies have shown that manipulating cholesterol metabolism inhibits tumor growth, reshapes the immunological landscape, and reinvigorates antitumor immune function.[20] Cholesterol is not found in plant food, only in animal food, and eggs are the highest source. The simplest way to eliminate excess cancer-fueling, immune-suppressing cholesterol in your body is to stop eating animal food. Your liver makes all the cholesterol you need.

IGF-1

Insulin-like growth factor-1 (IGF-1) is a growth hormone directly linked to uncontrolled cancer growth. In humans, elevated levels of IGf-1 can promote cancer, specifically breast, prostate, pancreatic, and colon cancer.[21] IGF-1 levels increase in your body when you eat animal protein and/or refined sugar. One remarkable study found that after just 12 days on a whole-food plant-based diet plus daily exercise, the blood of breast cancer patients was found to have significantly lower levels of IGF-1 and increased cancer-stopping power.[22]

Methionine

Many human cancer cells, including colorectal, breast, ovarian, melanoma, and leukemia, are dependent on an amino acid called methionine, which is one of nine amino acids not made by the body.[23,24] Fruits contain little to no methionine. Vegetables, nuts, and whole grains have small amounts. Beans have the most methionine in the plant kingdom; however, milk, eggs, and red meat have more than twice the methionine as beans, and chicken and fish have five to seven times more. The easiest way to keep your methionine levels low and deprive cancer cells of this essential amino acid is to eat little to no animal food.

Heme Iron

Heme iron is a highly absorbable form of iron found in meat—especially red meat, organ meat, and shellfish—but not in plant food. In small amounts, iron is good for you and necessary for the formation of healthy blood cells, but excess iron causes oxidative stress and DNA damage and can catalyze formation of cancer-causing N-nitroso compounds. Excess dietary iron has been linked to an increased risk of esophageal, stomach, colorectal, and breast cancer.[25,26,27] Excess iron accumulates in your liver, heart, and pancreas, eventually resulting in iron toxicity because your body has no way of ridding itself of excess iron except through blood loss. Non-heme iron is a much safer form of iron found in plant foods, especially in legumes, sesame seeds, pumpkin seeds, spinach, Swiss chard, quinoa, and dried apricots.

Neu5Gc

N-glycolylneuraminic acid (Neu5Gc) is a unique sugar molecule found only in animal food, especially red meat, organ meat, and some dairy products, which increases the risk of tumor formation in humans. Neu5Gc does not occur in humans. Your immune system treats this molecule as a foreign invader and produces antibodies in response to it; those antibodies increase inflammation in your body. Neu5Gc has been associated with inflammatory diseases including cancer, cardiovascular disease, and some bacterial infections.[28,29]

HCAs and PAHs

Cooking meat creates mutagenic compounds called heterocyclic amines (HCAs) and polycyclic aromatic hydrocarbons (PAHs). These are cancer-causing chemicals formed when muscle or organ meat and fat are cooked at high temperatures, as in barbecuing, baking, pan-frying, or grilling over an open flame. HCAs and PAHs are linked to various cancers, including kidney, colorectal, lung, prostate, and pancreatic cancer.[30,31,32,33,34]

One large study found that people with the highest consumption of meat cooked at high temperatures had a 70 percent greater risk of pancreatic cancer compared to those with the lowest consumption of well-done meats.[35] Fried bacon and fried fish have the highest concentrations of HCAs and PAHs, about five times more than beef and chicken. Interestingly, chicken cooked without the skin has been found to have twice the levels of mutagens as chicken cooked with the skin on.

Haven't humans been eating animals for thousands of years?
Yes, but not at the excessive levels that we do today. Thanks to the Industrial Revolution and factory farming, we are eating meat and/or dairy at nearly every meal. This seems normal, but it is unprecedented in human history, as are our rates of chronic diseases like cancer, heart disease, and diabetes. There are still many parts of the world

where cancer rates are very low. For example, the rate of colon cancer is 50 times lower in native Africans than in African Americans. Researchers credit the native Africans' extraordinarily low rates of colon cancer to an absence of "aggressive dietary factors," namely animal protein and fat.[36]

What about grass-fed, organic, wild meats?

When it comes to eating animal products, quality matters, but so does quantity. According to the National Geographic Blue Zones Project, the healthiest, longest-living people groups around the world eat diets that are 95 percent plant-based on average. This equates to eating animal products a few times per week, as opposed to two to three times per day. That is a much safer level of consumption for longevity promotion and disease prevention. If you choose to eat animal foods, I suggest a high-quality, low-quantity approach.

However, if you are trying to heal active cancer, I suggest applying the *precautionary principle* and reducing your consumption of animal products and processed foods to zero or near zero. Think in terms of risk reduction. When you reduce or eliminate the animal products in your diet and replace them with whole plant foods from the earth, you not only reduce the levels of cancer causers and cancer promoters found in animal food, but you also increase the levels of thousands of anticancer compounds found only in plant food. That's why a whole-food plant-based diet (organic as much as possible) is the optimal anticancer diet.

TO BEAN OR NOT TO BEAN

There's a lot of misinformation in the health and wellness space that creates unnecessary food fear. One of the most egregious examples of late is the demonization of legumes and whole grains. Legumes (beans, split peas, chickpeas, and lentils) are rich in vitamins, minerals, fiber, and prebiotic starch, and contain an essential anticancer compound called inositol hexaphosphate (IP6), also known as phytic acid, or phytates. IP6 is an antioxidant and has been found to reduce cancer cell proliferation and contribute to tumor cell destruction. It's even been shown to enhance the anticancer effects of chemotherapy, control cancer metastases, and improve quality of life for patients.[37]

Legumes along with many other vegetables and grains contain lectins, potentially problematic compounds that can interfere with the absorption of some nutrients, like minerals, but this effect is inactivated when lectins are cooked or soaked overnight. It's important to look at the big picture. If lectin-containing legumes were as harmful as some have claimed, they would not have the designation of being the food group most associated with longevity. It's true! The longest-living people groups on every continent of planet Earth consume the most legumes.[38]

Beans are delicious. They are a wonderful source of protein, fiber, and anticancer nutrients. They fill you up, satisfy you, and serve you well. Aim for one to three servings of legumes every day. Dried legumes are better than canned and can be prepared much more quickly than traditional methods by using a pressure cooker or an Instant Pot. But canned beans are still better than no beans.

Whole grains are also associated with longevity and low rates of chronic disease. They contain a wonderful assortment of vitamins, minerals, and phytonutrients including B vitamins, minerals, beta-glucans, phytates, and fiber. There are many whole grains to choose from and enjoy, but for simplicity's sake the recipes in this cookbook mainly feature whole grains that are gluten-free, easy to prepare, and don't require milling into flour.

ARSENIC IN RICE

It's estimated that 30,000 tons of arsenic-based weed killers were sprayed on cotton fields in the southern United States before being completely banned in the 1990s. As a result, rice grown in the South has high levels of arsenic compared to rice grown in other parts of the country, like California, and other parts of the world. Fortunately, there are numerous compounds in plant food that protect your cells, neutralize threats, bind to toxins, and help your body eliminate harmful toxins.

Studies have shown that curcumin, a compound in turmeric, binds to heavy metals like arsenic and lead and even reverses DNA damage caused by arsenic. Another study found that people with high levels of beta-carotene in the blood from eating foods like carrots, beets, sweet potatoes, and leafy greens had 99 percent lower odds of getting arsenic-induced cancer.[39,40] Based on these and numerous other protective factors that a diverse whole-food plant-based diet provides, we don't see arsenic in rice as a threat.

You will never be able to eat a perfectly clean, toxin-free diet—even if you grow every single thing you eat. The beautiful thing is that plants contain a wide variety of compounds that help protect you from the toxic stuff you can't avoid. Having said that, there are a few practical ways to reduce your exposure to arsenic in rice. Avoid rice grown in the southern United States. Limit rice consumption to a few times per week. And if you boil rice instead of steaming it, you can reduce the arsenic content by up to 60 percent. Rice substitutes include barley, farro, cauliflower rice, and chickpea rice.

A PINCH OF SALT

Sodium is a vital mineral for health and makes pretty much everything taste better, but there's a sweet spot when it comes to salt; too much or too little can be problematic. A sodium deficiency can cause hyponatremia, which in extreme cases can lead to coma and even death. On the flip side, excessive sodium is toxic to the body and injures your blood vessels, raises your blood pressure, and increases your risk of cardiovascular disease, kidney disease, and stomach cancer.[41] Excess sodium also suppresses the activity of one of your most important detoxification enzymes (superoxide dismutase)[42] and even weakens certain aspects of your immune system.[43]

The Western diet is dangerously high in sodium and the two biggest sources are processed food and restaurant food. Salt is a wonderful flavor enhancer, but it's best to use a pinch at the table rather than using large amounts in cooking. You'll end up consuming just the right amount of salt that way. In addition, deliberately using little to no salt for a few weeks resensitizes your taste buds to the subtle and complex flavors of food.

We use naturally harvested unprocessed salts such as sea salt or pink Himalayan salt; they have a mild, natural saltiness and contain trace minerals like magnesium, potassium, and calcium, which are stripped out of table salt. Naturally harvested salts are typically larger grained, comparable in size to kosher salt. They have less sodium by weight and are easier to pinch and spread over food. Taste a little bit of natural unprocessed salt side by side with table salt and you'll never go back to table salt. For simplicity's sake, sea salt is the type of salt listed in our recipes.

COOKING WITH GAS?

Gas ovens and cooktops produce air pollutants, namely carbon monoxide (CO) and nitrogen dioxide (NO_2), which is also found in car exhaust. A major study found that children who live in a home with a gas stove have a 42 percent higher risk of asthma symptoms and a 24 percent increased risk of being diagnosed with asthma.[44] NO_2 has been identified as a contributor to respiratory, cardiovascular, and immune system dysfunction and deterioration.[45] This is an easily avoidable toxin. When using a gas stove or cooktop, always turn the ventilation hood on.

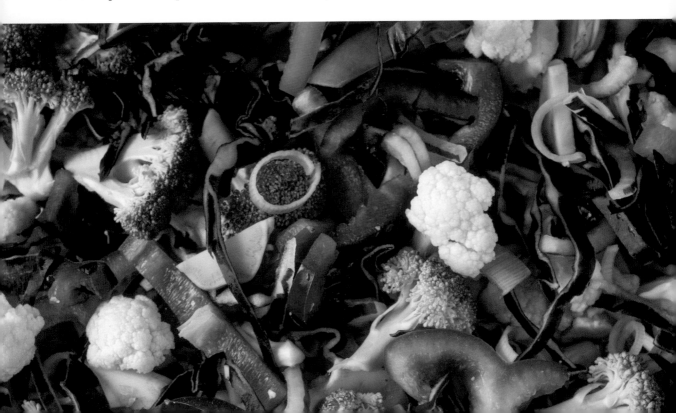

PANTRY STAPLES

Dried and canned beans (black, garbanzo, pinto, navy, etc.)
Dried lentils (black, red, green)
Oats
Quinoa
Rice (black, red, brown)
Almonds, walnuts, pecans, cashews, Brazil nuts, pine nuts, pepitas, etc.
Nut butters (almond, cashew, walnut, peanut, etc.)
Tahini
Flaxseeds
Chia seeds
Sunflower seeds
Hemp hearts
Apricots
Figs
Dates
Goji berries
Mulberries
Golden berries
Black currants
Raisins
Vegetable broth
Extra-virgin olive oil
Sesame oil
Coconut oil

IN THE SPICE RACK

Garlic powder
Turmeric
Curry powder
Cayenne pepper
Oregano
Cinnamon
Cumin
Allspice
Nutmeg
Thyme
Chili powder
Red pepper flakes
Bragg Organic Sprinkle
Harissa
Chinese five-spice powder
Vanilla extract
Sea salt or naturally harvested salt

SWEETENERS

Blackstrap molasses
Date sugar
Maple syrup
Honey (local or manuka)

IN THE FRIDGE

Apple cider vinegar
Tamari*
Coconut aminos**
Mustard
Horseradish
Pickles, sauerkraut, and/or kimchi
Plant milk (almond, cashew, oat, soy)
Cold-pressed flax oil

ESSENTIAL KITCHEN TOOLS

High-powered blender
Juicer
Garlic roller and press
Lemon squeezer
Coffee/seed grinder

*Tamari is a gluten-free soy sauce with less than a third of the sodium as traditional soy sauce.

**Coconut aminos is a soy-free, wheat-free, gluten-free alternative to soy sauce made from coconut tree sap and sea salt. It has 73 percent less sodium than soy sauce or liquid aminos and a similar savory but sweeter flavor. We love it!

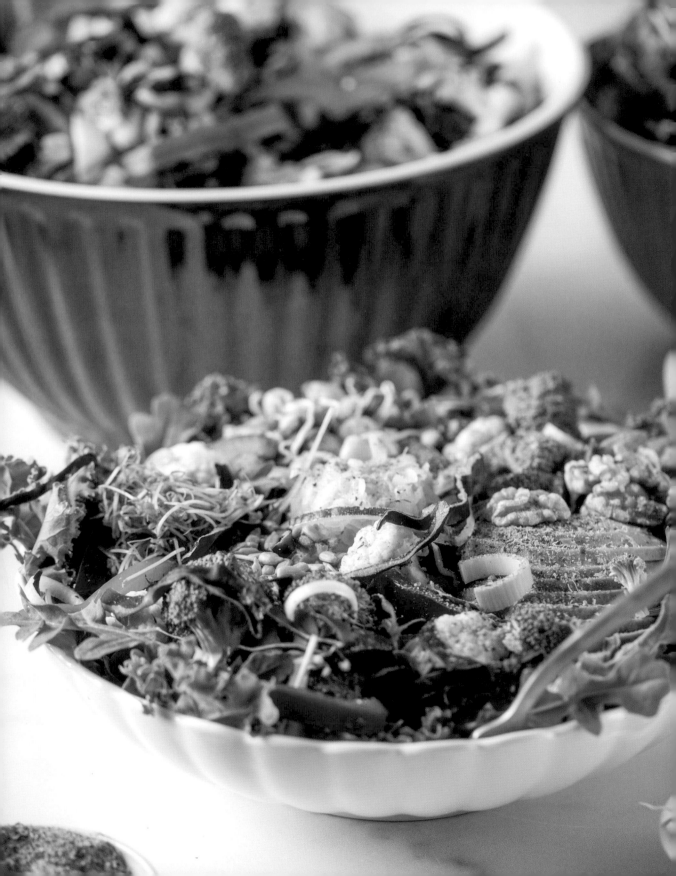

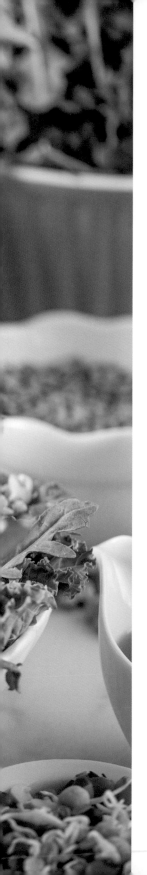

Part I

RECIPES FOR HEALING

In January 2004, in order to help my body heal stage IIIc colon cancer after surgery and in lieu of chemotherapy I chose to radically change my diet and "overdose on nutrition" with a 100 percent organic, raw, plant-based diet. After experimenting with various raw food recipes, I realized that the most nutritionally dense and diverse anticancer meal I could eat was a giant salad, so that became my default meal for lunch and dinner.

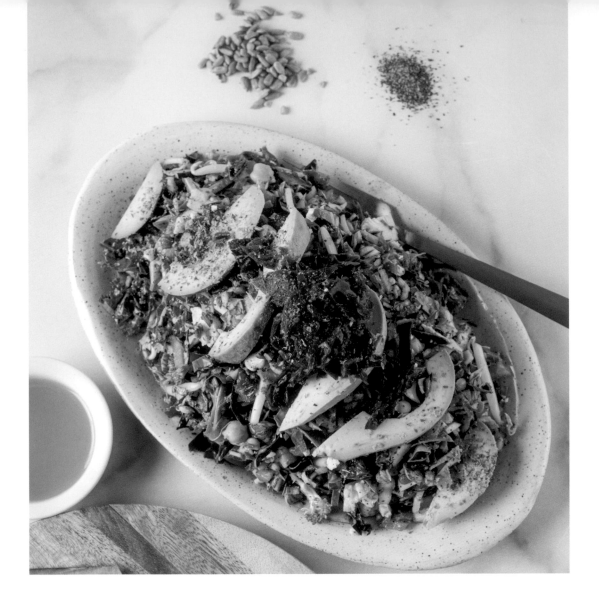

I ate the Giant Cancer-Fighting Salad every day because I didn't want to sacrifice nutritional potency for the sake of variety—and because it was simple, sustainable, delicious, and efficient. The Giant Salad is the ultimate fast food. You just toss the ingredients into a bowl and eat! Once I got into the groove, I knew exactly how much produce to buy at the grocery store each week. There's no menu planning required, and no food is wasted. You eat everything you buy. And that's a good feeling too.

One of my favorite nutritional science studies happened in 2009. Researchers dripped 34 fresh vegetable juices onto eight different types of cancer cells and found that nearly every vegetable from the allium and cruciferous families completely stopped cancer growth.[46] The top three most powerful anticancer vegetables were all from the allium family: garlic, leeks, and onions. Right behind those were the cruciferous veggies broccoli, cauliflower, kale, and cabbage. These are the staple ingredients of my Giant Salad!

The cruciferous family also includes cancer-fighters arugula, watercress, Brussels sprouts, bok choy, collard greens, radishes, turnips, kohlrabi, mustard, horseradish, and wasabi. Other noteworthy anticancer veggies from this study are beetroot, asparagus, green beans, rutabaga, and hot peppers.

Many of the top anticancer veggies like garlic, onions, leeks, broccoli, cauliflower, kale, and cabbage are best consumed raw as cooking destroys enzymes, kills beneficial bacteria, and reduces the potency and availability of specific anticancer nutrients found in these vegetables, including allicin in garlic and sulforaphane in crucifers.

Research has repeatedly shown that the most effective, evidence-based anticancer diet is one that contains at least 10 servings of fruits and vegetables per day. One Giant Salad is about four to five servings of vegetables. Two salads per day gets you right around 10 servings. And that doesn't even count breakfast, snacks, or juicing.

The Giant Cancer-Fighting Salad is the simplest, most sustainable, most potent anticancer meal possible. And it was an integral part of my healing strategy.

If you are serious about healing cancer or preventing a recurrence, keep it simple and follow the recipes in Part I. Have a smoothie or oatmeal for breakfast; eat the Giant Salad for lunch and dinner; and drink 40 to 64 ounces of fresh vegetable juice every day between and with meals. That will put you in the ideal anticancer range of 15 to 20 servings of fruits and vegetables per day.

And chew your food well. The better you chew, the more nutrients you absorb!

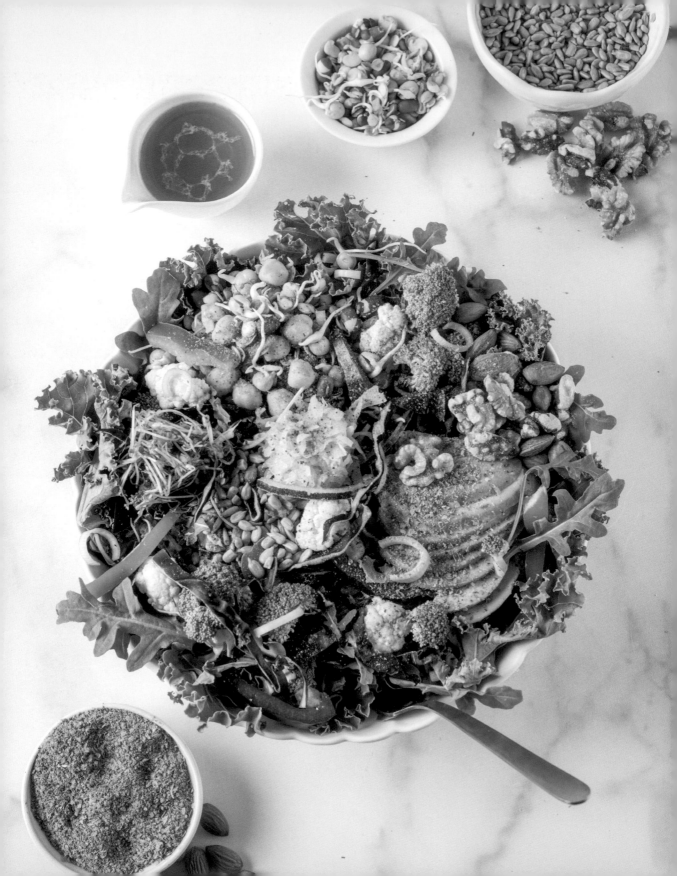

GIANT CANCER-FIGHTING SALAD

Serves 1 to 2

1 handful of leafy greens:
kale, spinach, Swiss chard,
watercress, arugula

1 handful of broccoli

1 handful of cauliflower

½ leek, sliced, washed,
and rinsed in a colander

1 to 3 purple cabbage leaves,
torn into smaller pieces

1 red, yellow, or green pepper,
sliced

1 to 2 slices red, yellow,
or green onion

½ avocado, sliced

1 handful of raw, unsalted
almonds or walnuts, whole
or chopped

1 to 3 tablespoons sunflower
seeds

1 to 3 tablespoons hemp
seeds

½ cup legumes, sprouted
(garbanzo beans, lentils,
mung beans) or cooked
(black, garbanzo, kidney
beans, etc.)

¼ cup sauerkraut or Ruby
Kraut (page 199)

¼ cup Broccoli Sprouts
(page 20)

Anticancer Vinaigrette
(recipe follows), to taste

Super Sofrito (page 204),
to taste

Anticancer Sprinkle
(recipe follows), to taste

1. Spread the leafy greens in a single layer on the bottom of a large bowl.

2. Add the broccoli, cauliflower, leek, cabbage, pepper, and onion.

3. Top with the avocado, nuts, sunflower seeds, hemp seeds, legumes, sauerkraut, and broccoli sprouts.

4. Season with Anticancer Salad Sprinkle, Super Sofrito (page 204), or spices of your choice and drizzle with the Anticancer Vinaigrette.

NOTE: If you haven't made the Anticancer Sprinkle yet, you can just shake on the spices individually.

All vegetables are wonderful. Feel free to add any others you like. Availability and pricing will vary based on the season. Also, soaking and sprouting unlocks enzymes and nutrition in nuts and seeds and may make them easier to digest, but this is not mandatory. Unsprouted nuts and seeds are wonderful healthy foods as well. Legumes should be soaked and sprouted if consumed raw. Otherwise, cook them.

ANTICANCER VINAIGRETTE

This salad dressing is customizable to your taste. Drizzle and sprinkle the ingredients to get the balance you like.

Extra-virgin olive oil and/or flaxseed oil

Apple cider vinegar

Oregano

Garlic powder

Turmeric or curry powder

Cayenne pepper

Black pepper

Bragg Organic Sprinkle

Nutritional yeast

Lightly drizzle the oil and apple cider vinegar to taste. Then shake on the spices and toss the salad. Go easy on the cayenne at first; it's spicy. If you don't like the taste of apple cider vinegar, lemon juice is a great addition or substitute. Feel free to experiment with ingredients to create your perfect blend.

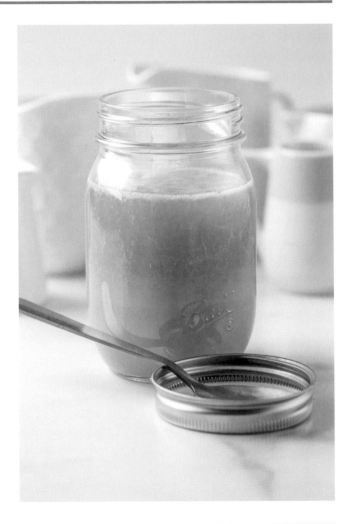

Oil on salad increases the absorption of fat-soluble vitamins and micronutrients. Fresh-pressed olive oil contains the highest levels of a unique anticancer compound called oleocanthol.[47] Flaxseeds contain anticancer lignans and are among the highest sources of anti-inflammatory omega-3 alpha linolenic acid in the plant kingdom. One tablespoon of flax oil contains three times as much omega-3s as a tablespoon of ground flax.

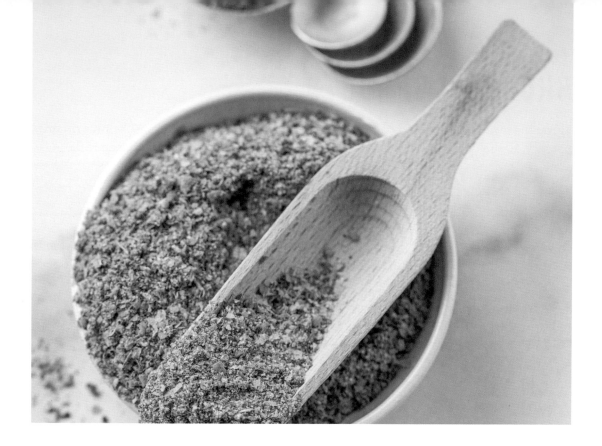

ANTICANCER SPRINKLE

Here's how to premix the anticancer spices to save time. This also makes a great seasoning for cooked veggies. Enjoy!

Yield: About ½ cup

1 tablespoon dried oregano

1 teaspoon granulated garlic or garlic powder

1 tablespoon curry powder or turmeric

¼ teaspoon cayenne pepper

1 teaspoon black pepper

2 tablespoons mixed seasoning, such as Italian seasoning or Bragg Organic Sprinkle, or both

2 tablespoons nutritional yeast

Place all the ingredients in a small Mason jar or resealable container and shake until they are well mixed. You can keep this mixture in your spice cabinet and put it on everything.

BROCCOLI SPROUTS

Sprouting legumes, seeds, nuts, and grains brings them to life and increases their nutritional potency. Here's how to grow broccoli sprouts (the process is essentially the same for all sprouts).

1 tablespoon of broccoli seeds yields about 2 cups of sprouts.

1. Soak the broccoli seeds overnight in filtered water in a Mason jar with a screen lid.

2. On day 2, drain the water, rinse the seeds with filtered water, and drain again.

3. Rinse the seeds twice per day for 4 to 5 days. When the tail on the sprout is about an inch long, they're ready to eat.

4. Store in the fridge for up to 7 to 10 days.

PRO TIPS:

- To keep a fresh supply of sprouts, start a new batch a day or 2 after your first batch is ready to eat.

- Sprouting jars and sprouting trays make this process even easier. You can find them at health food stores and online.

- Freezing broccoli sprouts increases their sulforaphane content by $1\frac{1}{2}$ to 2 times.[48] I suggest blending frozen broccoli sprouts into a smoothie.

- Dried chickpeas, green lentils, and mung beans also make great sprouts.

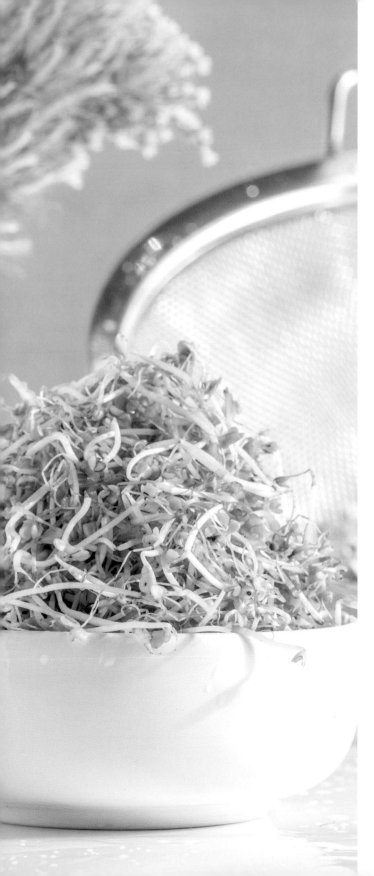

Your body's first line of defense against pathogens, bacteria, viruses, parasites, and cancer-causing toxins are intestinal immune cells called intraepithelial lymphocytes. These cells are covered in special receptors that are activated by indole-3-carbinol in broccoli and other cruciferous veggies, essentially supercharging them. Broccoli also contains an anticancer compound called sulforaphane, which is the most potent phase 2 liver detoxification enzyme known and is created by a chemical reaction that happens when you chop or chew raw broccoli. Cruciferous veggies are most potent when consumed raw, but if you plan to cook them, chop them and allow them to sit for 40 minutes before cooking to allow the sulforaphane reaction to take place. You can also add mustard powder to cooked cruciferous veggies to facilitate this chemical reaction.

Broccoli sprouts contain roughly 25 times more sulforaphane and 100 times more indole-3-carbinol than mature broccoli, and they can be found in the refrigerated produce section of most grocery stores right next to the alfalfa sprouts. You can also purchase broccoli seeds and sprout them in three to four days at home, which makes them the cheapest and most powerful immune-boosting and detoxifying medicinal food on Earth. Broccoli sprouts should be eaten raw and are great on salads.

Please note that it is possible to get too much of a good thing. Too much sulforaphane could make you feel sick, so it's recommended that you do not eat more than four cups of broccoli sprouts per day. Two to three cups per day should keep you on the safe side.

CANCER-FIGHTING SOUP

I ate my Giant Cancer-Fighting Salad every day for lunch and dinner for several years. It truly is the most potent anticancer meal. Your digestive system will adapt to eating large amounts of raw vegetables, but it takes time, typically no more than a week or two. I understand that some folks have unique dietary challenges. To help with the transition and to break up the monotony, we created two super-delicious variations of the Giant Cancer-Fighting Salad for you: a soup and a sheet-pan bake. Gently cooking the veggies preserves their nutrients while making them easier to digest. It's also nice if you are craving warm food in cold winter months.

Yield: 10 to 12 cups | *Serves 4 to 6*

4 cups Juicer Broth (page 214)

2 cups water

2 cups broccoli, chopped

1 cup cauliflower, chopped

2 cups baby kale or spinach

1 cup red or purple cabbage, chopped

2 celery ribs, diced

4 garlic cloves, minced

3 mushrooms, sliced

1 red bell pepper, diced

½ red onion, diced

1 leek, halved lengthwise, light green and white parts sliced

1½ cups cooked chickpeas or one 15-ounce can of chickpeas, drained and rinsed

1 tablespoon Anticancer Sprinkle (page 19)

2 teaspoons apple cider vinegar

Toppings

Avocado, sliced

Almonds, chopped

Walnuts, chopped

Sunflower seeds

Sauerkraut or kimchi

1. Place all the ingredients in a stockpot and bring to a boil, stirring occasionally.

2. Reduce the heat, cover, and simmer for 5 minutes.

3. Ladle the soup into bowls and top each with ½ sliced avocado and garnish with almonds, walnuts, sunflower seeds, and sauerkraut.

Feel free to use additional Anticancer Sprinkle or any other spice you enjoy. And don't leave out the sauerkraut or kimchi—they really make this soup pop!

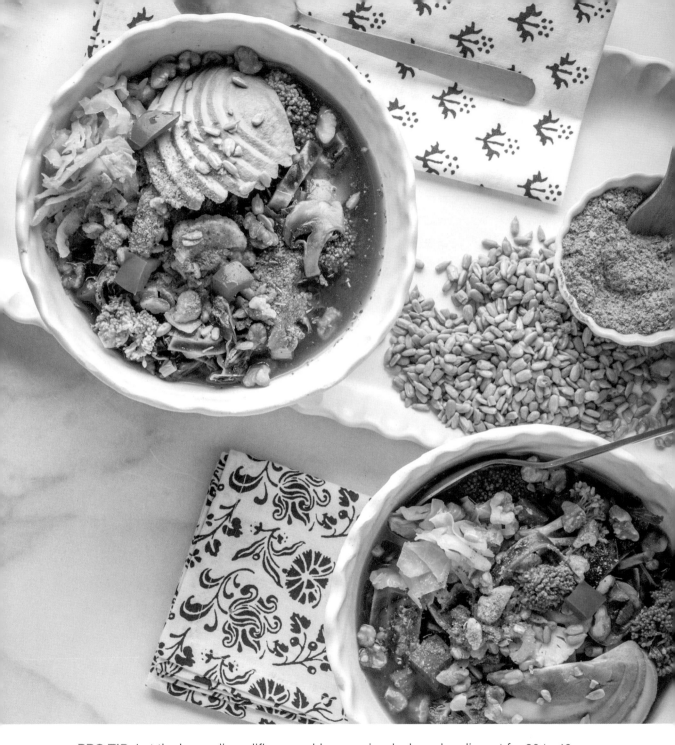

PRO TIP: Let the broccoli, cauliflower, cabbage, onion, leek, and garlic rest for 20 to 40 minutes after chopping and before cooking to maximize the formation of anticancer compounds like sulforaphane.

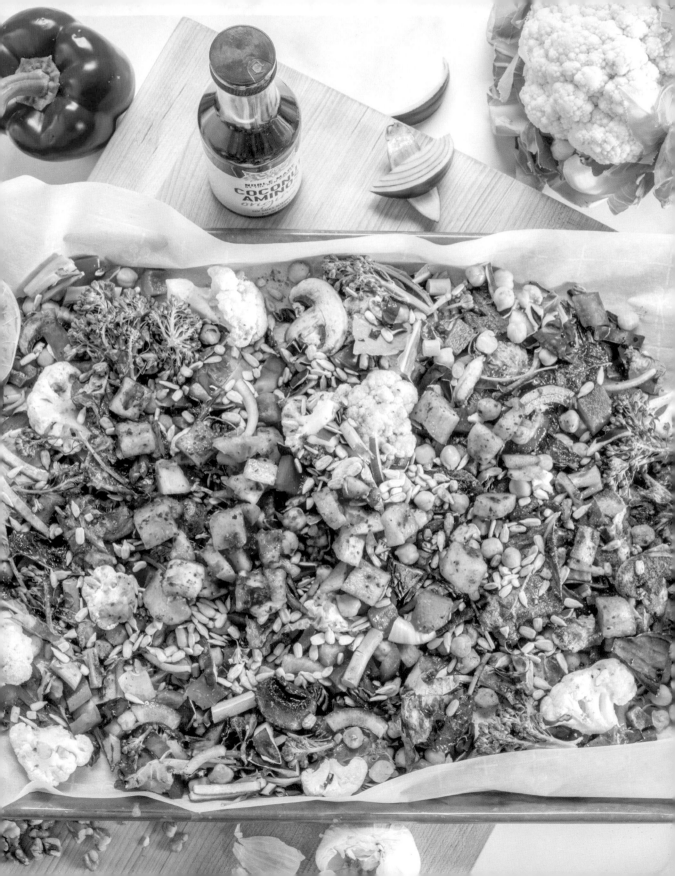

CANCER-FIGHTING SHEET-PAN BAKE

Yield: 10 to 12 cups | *Serves 4 to 6*

2 to 3 cups broccoli florets

2 cups cauliflower florets

1 cup chopped red or purple cabbage

1 red bell pepper, diced

3 mushrooms, sliced

½ red onion, sliced

1½ cups cooked chickpeas or one 15-ounce can chickpeas, drained and rinsed

2 cups baby kale or spinach

2 tablespoons olive oil

1 tablespoon Anticancer Sprinkle (page 19)

6 garlic cloves, minced

¼ cup sauerkraut or kimchi

⅛ cup sunflower seeds

¼ cup sliced almonds or walnuts, to garnish

Coconut aminos, to drizzle

1 cup cooked rice or quinoa (optional)

1. Preheat your oven to 350 degrees.

2. Spread the broccoli, cauliflower, cabbage, bell pepper, mushrooms, onion, chickpeas, and kale in a single layer on a large, parchment-lined baking sheet. Drizzle the olive oil and spread the Anticancer Sprinkle and minced garlic evenly over the veggies, then bake for 15 minutes. The object is to wilt the greens and warm the vegetables without cooking them too much.

3. Garnish with sauerkraut, sunflower seeds, and nuts, drizzle with coconut aminos, add a side of rice, if desired, and serve.

PRO TIP: Let the broccoli, cauliflower, cabbage, onion, and garlic rest for 20 to 40 minutes after chopping and before cooking to maximize the formation of anticancer compounds like sulforaphane.

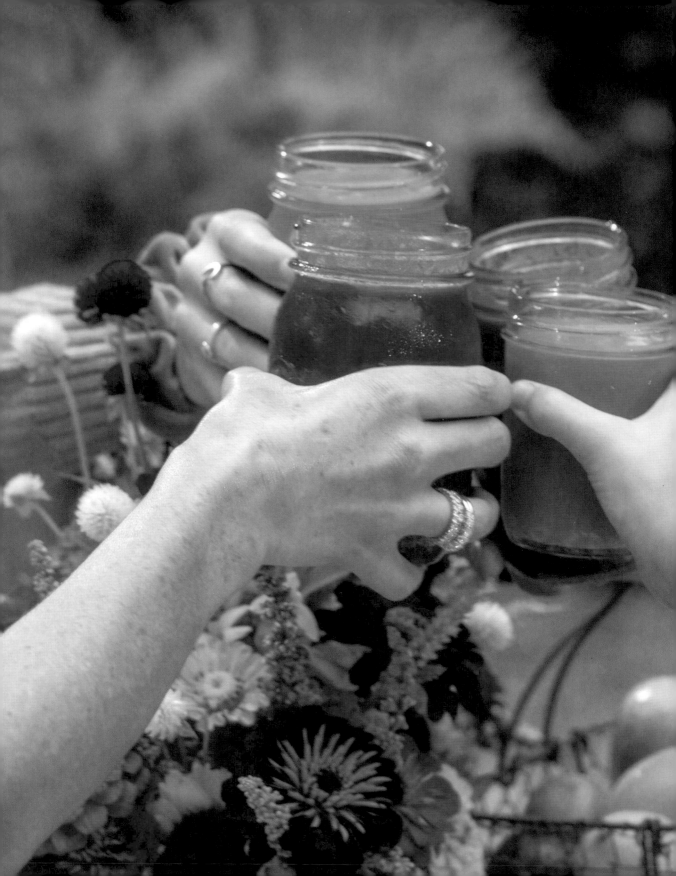

FRESH JUICES

Juicing vs. Blending

Juicing and *blending* are not interchangeable terms. Here's the difference: Juicing extracts juice from the fiber in produce. Blending blends it all together. You make juice with a juicer and smoothies with a blender. Neither juicing nor blending is better than the other because they serve different purposes. Blending fruits and veggies into a smoothie gives you a meal or a snack. The intention of juicing is to give you supplemental nutrition. Juicing is a way to get more nutrients (vitamins, minerals, enzymes, antioxidants, etc.) into your body in addition to what you are eating at meals. Juices can be consumed with and between meals.

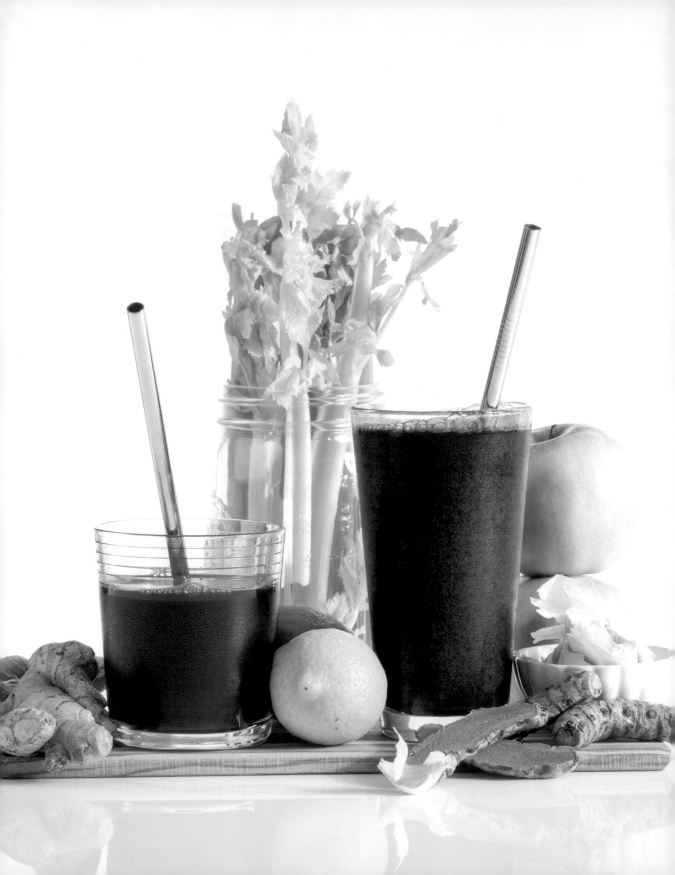

BASIC ANTICANCER JUICE FORMULA

Serves 1 to 2

5 small carrots

1 to 2 celery stalks

½ beetroot (and a few beet greens)

1-inch piece of fresh ginger

Juice all the ingredients together to determine how many ounces of juice your juicer yields. Then multiply the ingredients to get the desired amount of juice you want to make each day.

ADVANCED ANTICANCER JUICE FORMULA

Serves 1 to 2

5 small carrots

1 to 2 celery stalks

½ beetroot (and a few beet greens)

1- to 2-inch piece of gingerroot (or as much as you can stand)

1- to 2-inch piece of turmeric root (or as much as you can stand)

¼ to ½ lemon or lime, unpeeled

1 whole green apple, unpeeled

1 garlic clove (or as much as you can stand)

Juice all the ingredients together to determine how many ounces of juice your juicer yields. Then multiply the ingredients to get the desired amount of juice you want to make each day.

These additional ingredients may be added after the fact to amp up the nutritional value:

1 scoop greens powder

¼ to 1 teaspoon amla powder

¼ to 1 teaspoon moringa powder

½ teaspoon matcha green tea powder

2 to 6 ounces aloe vera gel

MERRY MARY

Move over Bloody Mary, our Merry Mary is a savory tomato-based juice packed with anticancer, antioxidant, and anti-inflammatory veggies: celery, pepper, jalapeño, carrots, and garlic. Enjoy this fun, festive juice anytime you like.

Yield: About 6 cups | *Serves 4 to 6*

1 pound tomatoes

1 celery stalk, plus small inner ribs for garnish

1 large cucumber

1 medium green bell pepper

4 medium carrots

1 garlic clove

1 medium jalapeño pepper (optional), plus more for garnish

2 medium limes, cut into wedges

Black pepper, to taste

4 to 6 pieces pickled okra

4 to 6 radishes

4 to 6 olives

4 to 6 grape tomatoes

1. Feed the tomatoes, celery, cucumber, bell pepper, carrots, garlic, and jalapeño, if using, into your juicer.

2. Transfer the juice to a 2-quart pitcher and stir together. Divide the juice among 4 to 6 glasses on ice.

3. Garnish with a lime wedge, a sprinkle of black pepper, a rib of celery, a piece of pickled okra, a radish, an olive, and a grape tomato.

Tomatoes contain a unique anticancer compound called lycopene. And high intake of tomatoes has been associated with a lower risk of multiple types of cancer including prostate, lung, stomach, colorectal, breast, and others.[49]

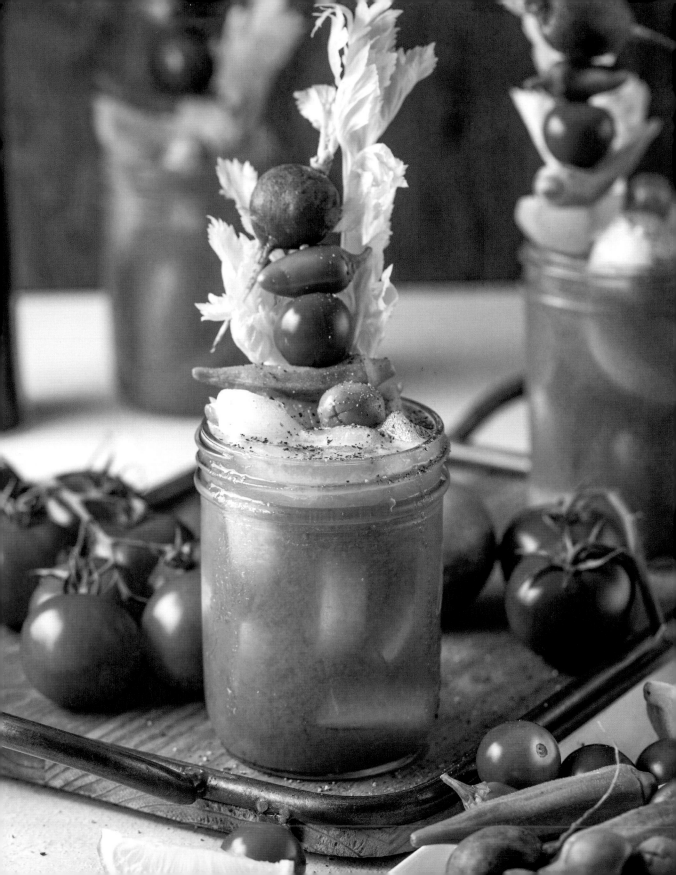

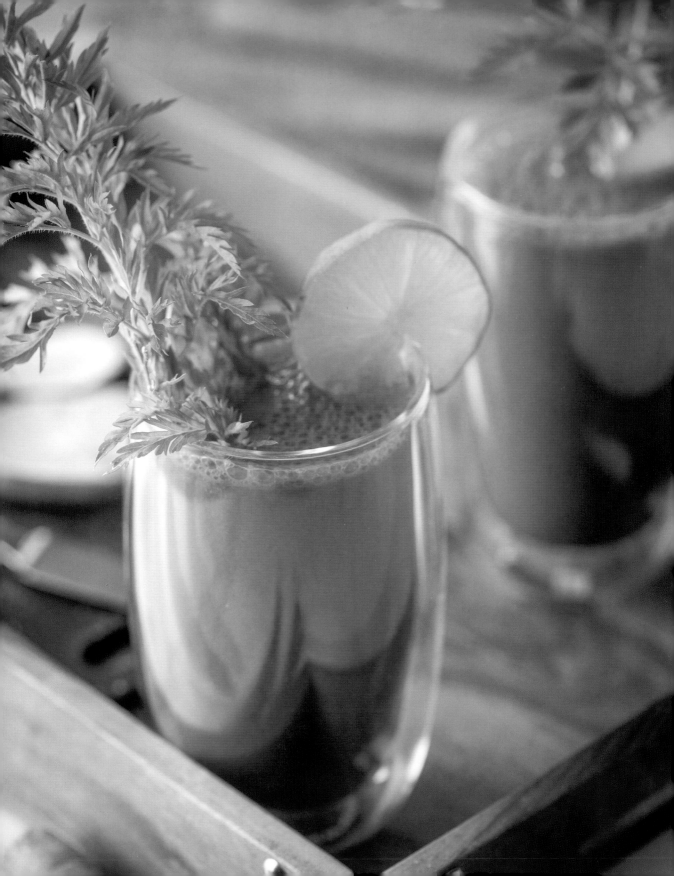

CARROT-LIME JUICE

Something magical happens when you combine carrot and lime juice that cannot be described. You'll just have to do it and see! This two-ingredient juice is super simple and so yummy that everyone in the family will love it.

Yield: 4 to 5 cups | *Serves 4*

---

5 pounds carrots, trimmed

3 limes, unpeeled

1. Feed the carrots and limes into your juicer.

2. Transfer the juice to a 2-quart pitcher and stir together; divide among 4 glasses.

PRO TIP: Freeze carrot pulp whenever you juice carrots to use in our Carrot Cake Pancakes page 52.

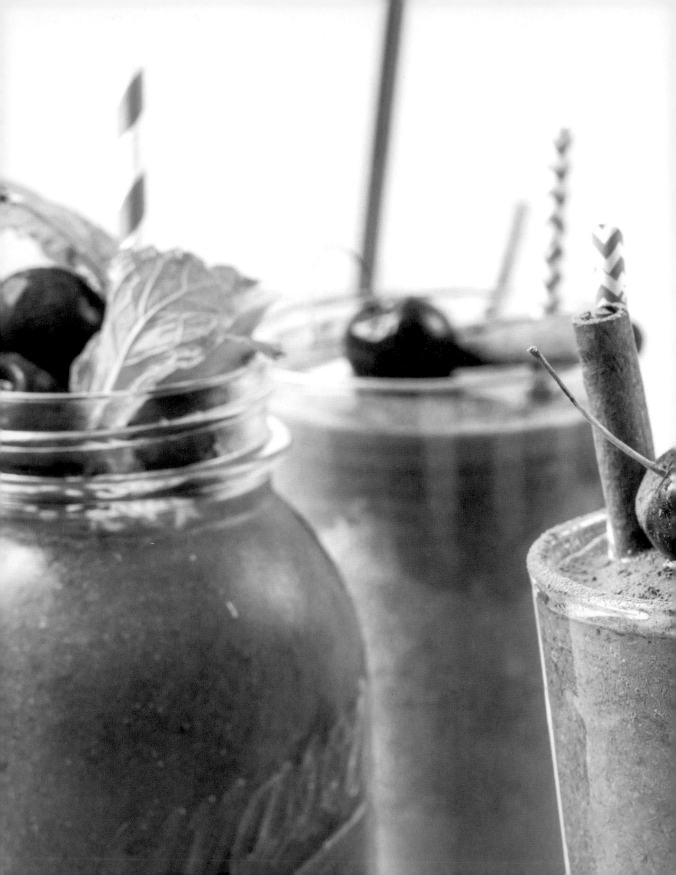

SMOOTHIES

Berries are the most potent anticancer fruits, and I love adding fresh berries to oatmeal and snacking on them by the handful. But it can be difficult to get organically grown berries, and they often get moldy quickly. The most practical and economical way to consume berries is to buy them frozen and blend them up in smoothies. Plus, using frozen ingredients negates the need for ice. A large smoothie can be a meal, and I love having one for breakfast or lunch. A small smoothie can be a snack or dessert. Enjoy!

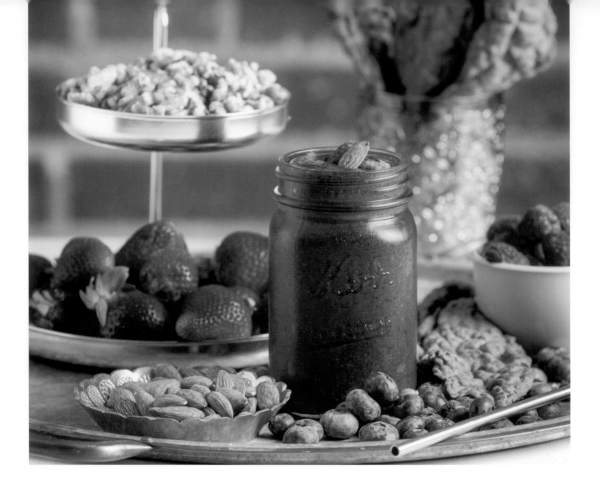

ANTICANCER SMOOTHIE

Yield: About 32 ounces | *Serves 1 to 2*

3 cups frozen mixed berries (blueberries, blackberries, raspberries, and/or strawberries)

1 banana, fresh or frozen, or 3 to 5 pitted dates

½ lemon, with peel

2 handfuls of leafy greens like spinach or kale

1 handful of almonds or walnuts, or both

1 cup water

Combine all the ingredients in your blender until smooth, adding another ½ cup of water if needed.

GREEN SMOOTHIE

Yield: About 32 ounces | *Serves 1 to 2*

3 cups baby kale

1 banana, fresh or frozen

1 cup frozen mango or frozen pineapple

1 cup frozen cherries

3 medium Medjool dates, pitted

1 to 2 tablespoons whole flaxseed or flax oil

¼ cup mint (optional)

1 to 1½ cups water

Place all the ingredients in your blender and combine until smooth, adding another ¹/₂ cup of water if needed.

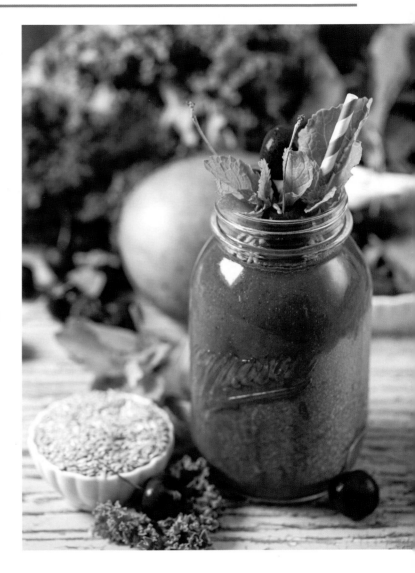

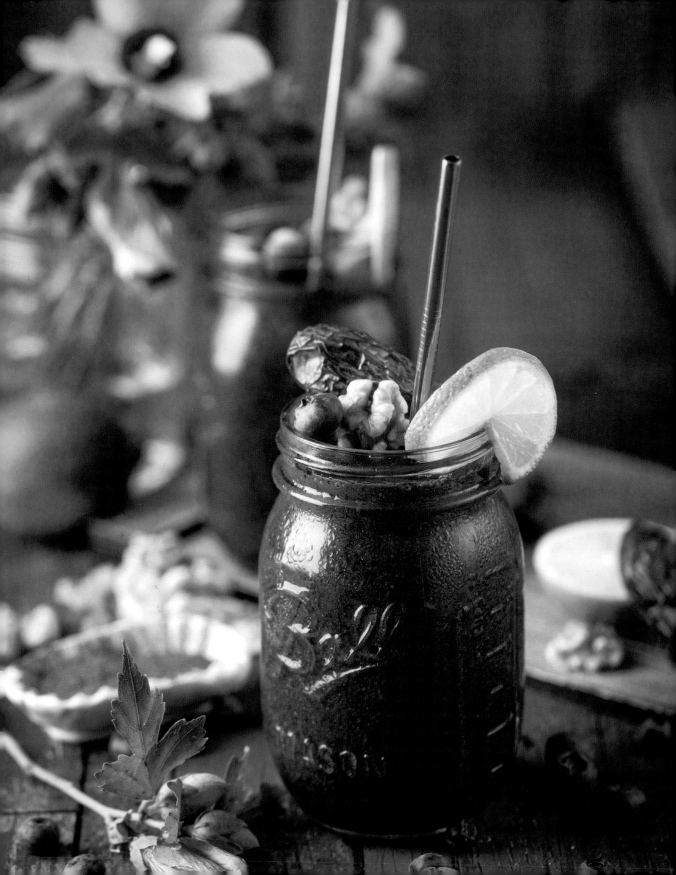

BLUEBERRY-LIME HIBISCUS SMOOTHIE

Yield: About 32 ounces | *Serves 1 to 2*

3 cups frozen blueberries

1 banana, fresh or frozen

½ teaspoon hibiscus powder

½ teaspoon moringa powder

¼ cup walnuts

2 medium Medjool dates, pitted

½ lime, unpeeled

1 to 1½ cups water

Place all the ingredients in your blender and combine until smooth, adding another ½ cup of water if needed.

Natural killer (NK) cells are a type of immune cell that fights viral infections and cancer cells. Blueberries boost your immune system by increasing the number of natural killer cells in your body![51]

CHERRY-CACAO SMOOTHIE

Yield: About 32 ounces | *Serves 1 to 2*

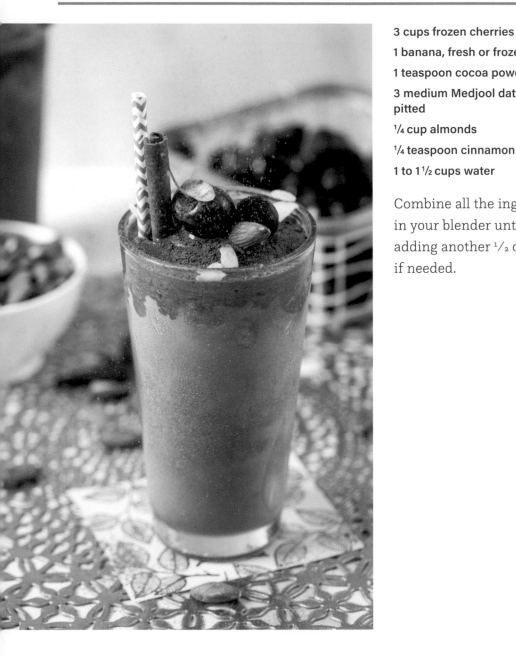

3 cups frozen cherries

1 banana, fresh or frozen

1 teaspoon cocoa powder

3 medium Medjool dates, pitted

¼ cup almonds

¼ teaspoon cinnamon

1 to 1½ cups water

Combine all the ingredients in your blender until smooth, adding another ½ cup of water if needed.

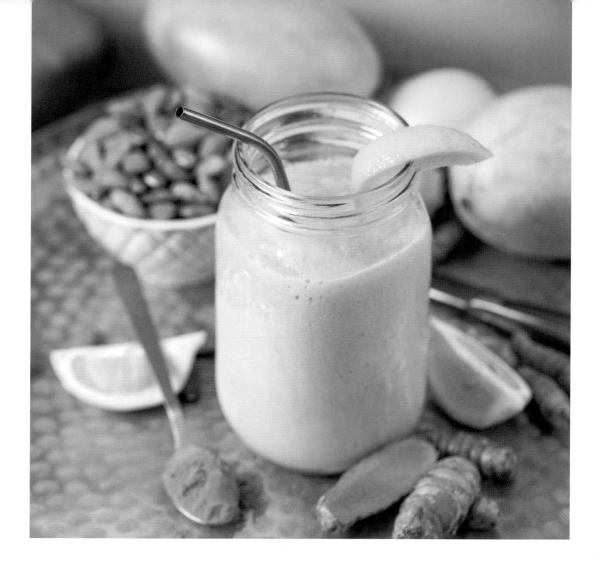

MANGO TURMERIC TART SMOOTHIE

Yield: About 32 ounces | *Serves 1 to 2*

2 cups frozen mango

2 medium frozen bananas

1 teaspoon turmeric powder

¼ organic lemon, with peel and seeds

¼ cup almonds

1 to 1½ cups water

Place all the ingredients in your blender and combine until smooth, adding another ½ cup of water if needed.

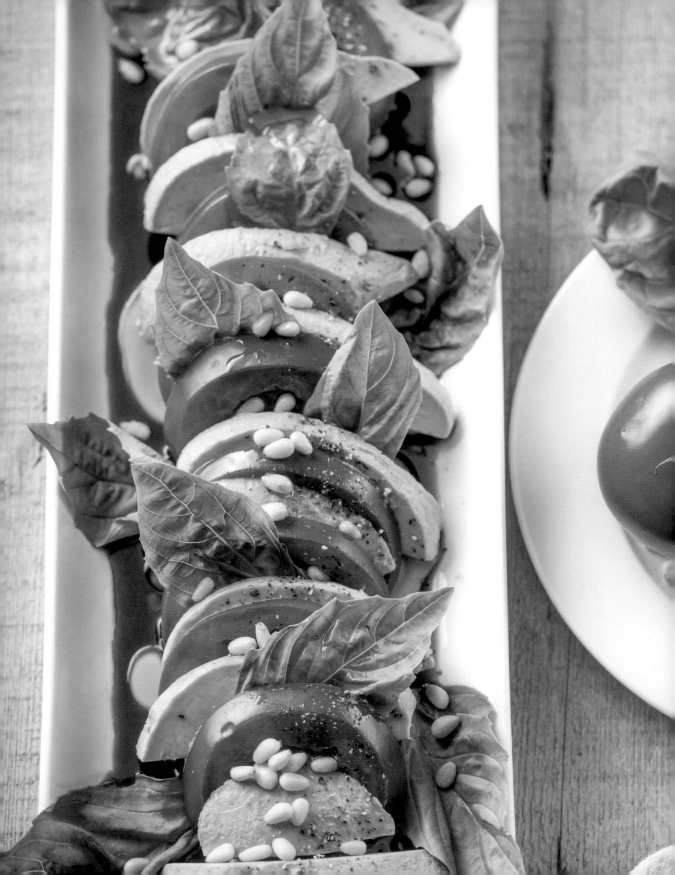

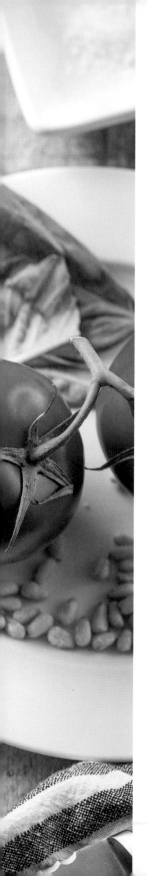

Part II

RECIPES FOR PREVENTION

If you live and eat the way everyone else does, you can expect to get the same chronic diseases everyone else gets.

During the most intensive healing phase of my cancer journey, I chose to eat the most potent anticancer foods every day. It was a simple routine of fresh juices, giant salads, and fruit smoothies. My diet was 100 percent raw food for the first 90 days. Then 80 percent raw from there. After several years of eating this hardcore anticancer diet, and once I was confident that I was out of the high-risk zone, my focus shifted from healing disease to eating for longevity. And that led me to branch out, explore, and experiment with new recipes. The whole-food plant-based recipes in this section represent the way we eat now. And after 17 years, I still love giant salads, smoothies, and fresh juices.

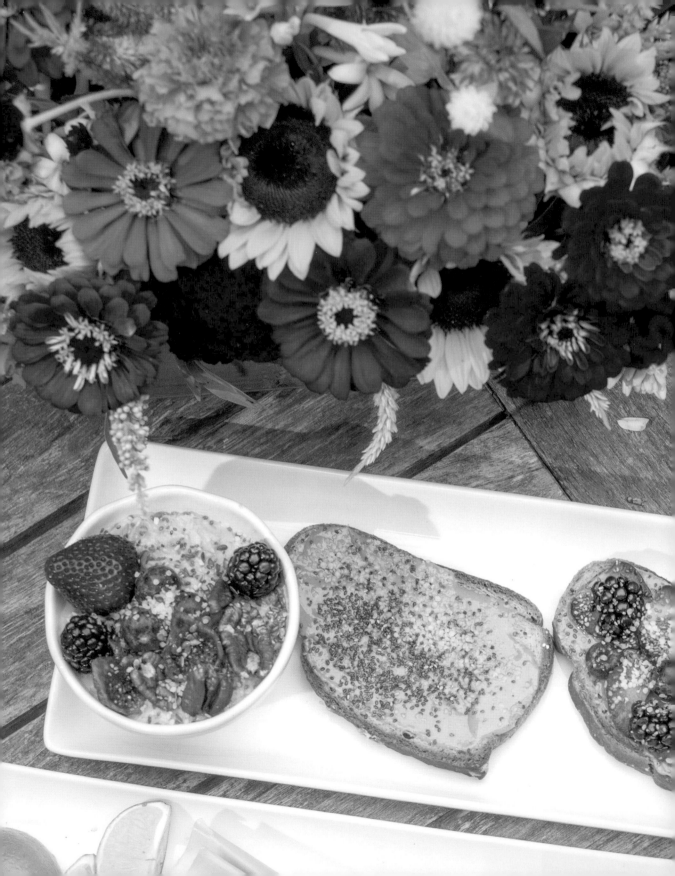

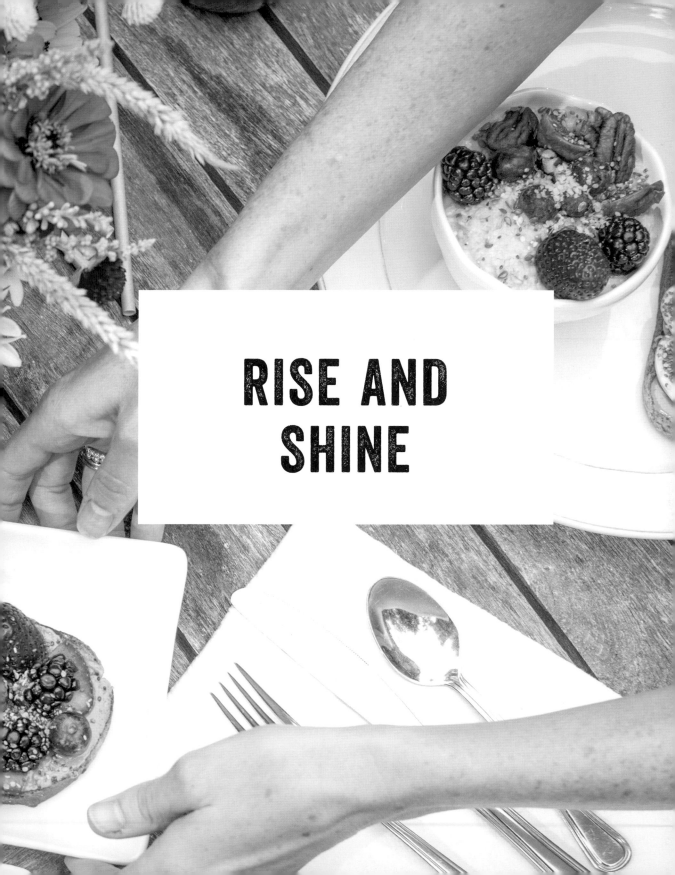

RISE AND SHINE

SUPERCHARGED OATMEAL

Our Supercharged Oatmeal is truly the breakfast of champions. It's my go-to breakfast at home and when I travel. Oatmeal is easy to make; it will fill you up and give you steady energy all morning, and you can make it a different way every day. The combinations of nuts, seeds, fruits, and spices you can add are endless. Buffet-style oatmeal is great for the family—that way everybody can pick their own toppings.

Yield: About 6 cups | *Serves 4*

2 cups rolled oats

2 cups almond milk

2 cups water

4 tablespoons ground flaxseeds

4 tablespoons whole or ground chia seeds

1 teaspoon cinnamon

¼ teaspoon allspice

Dried fruit options, such as black currants, goji berries, raisins, mulberries, sliced figs, or sliced apricots

Sweetener, such as blackstrap molasses or maple syrup, to taste

Fresh fruit toppings, such as blueberries, raspberries, strawberries, and bananas

Nut/seed toppings, such as almonds, walnuts, pecans, hemp hearts, pumpkin seeds, or a dollop of nut butter

1. Whisk together the oats, nut milk, water, flax, chia, cinnamon, allspice, and dried fruit of your choice in a medium pot over medium heat.

2. Cook until heated through and the mixture has thickened to your desired consistency, about 5 minutes.

3. Serve warm with your favorite toppings: sweetener, fresh fruit, nuts, and seeds.

PRO TIP: Flax and chia seeds can be quickly ground in a small coffee grinder before adding to oatmeal for maximum freshness and nutritional potency.

To make overnight oats, mix the core ingredients together in a covered bowl or Mason jar, refrigerate overnight, and enjoy cold or warmed up the next morning with fresh toppings.

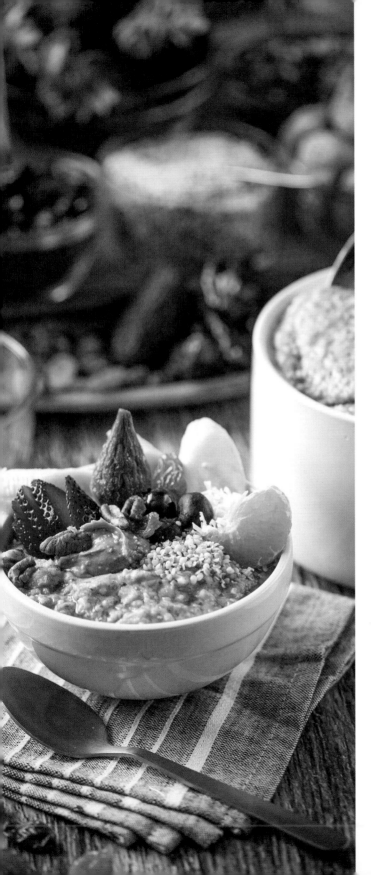

Which form of oats is best?

Oats come four ways: whole oat groats, steel-cut, rolled, and quick oats. Whole oat groats are the edible kernel of an oat with the hull removed, and they look a bit like a cross between a grain of rice and a grain of barley. Steel-cut oats are groats that have been chopped into two to three smaller pieces. Rolled oats are whole oat groats that have been steamed, rolled flat, and lightly toasted, which is why they cook faster, in about five minutes. Quick oats are rolled then chopped into smaller bits so they cook the most quickly, after just a couple of minutes in hot water.

The nutrient content among all forms of oats is essentially the same, but because they are precooked, the carbohydrates in rolled oats and quick oats are absorbed more quickly by your body and have been found to raise blood sugar and insulin about 30 percent more than whole oat groats and steel-cut oats.

Based on that, one could make the case that whole oat groats and steel-cut oats are "healthier," but I often opt for rolled or quick oats due to their superquick cook time. The most efficient way to prepare steel-cut oats is in a pressure cooker, which takes less than 30 minutes. You can also soak oats overnight in water or your favorite nut milk and serve them cold or warmed up on the stove.

A meta-analysis of 12 studies on nearly 800,000 people published by researchers at Harvard found that eating 70 grams of whole grains per day—that's a large bowl of oatmeal—lowers the risk of death from cancer and heart disease by 20 percent.[50]

JALAPEÑO STRAWBERRY AVOCADO TOAST

Our avocado toast starts with our Lemony Almond Hummus spread over sprouted whole-grain bread, then we layer sliced avocado, and top it with jalapeño and strawberries to add the perfect balance of heat and sweet. Super yum!

Yield: 4 slices | *Serves 4*

4 slices sprouted whole-grain bread

½ cup Lemony Almond Hummus (page 191)

1 medium jalapeño, thinly sliced

4 medium strawberries, sliced and tops removed

1 large Hass avocado, sliced

1 green onion, sliced

Sea salt and black pepper, to taste

1. Toast the bread slices to a golden brown.

2. Divide the hummus evenly among the slices of toast, then shingle alternating slices of jalapeño, strawberry, and avocado on top.

3. Garnish with green onion, salt, and pepper.

PRO TIP: Nearly all the heat in peppers is in the seeds, ribs, and membranes. If you prefer a milder jalapeño, simply slice the pepper lengthwise and use the top of your knife to scrape out the seeds and lighter-colored ribs and membranes, discarding those parts. Slice the remaining pepper to use in the recipe.

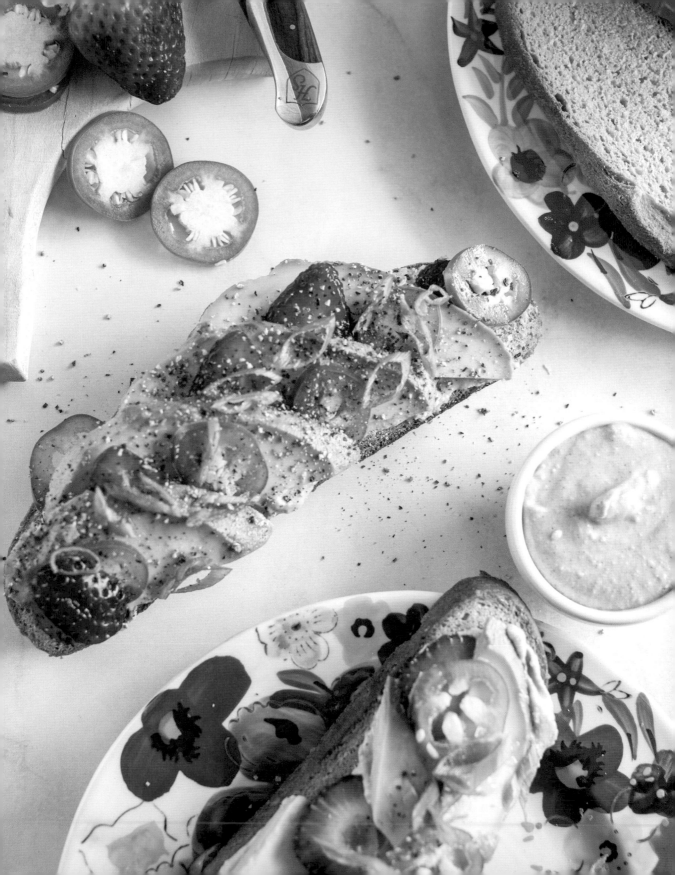

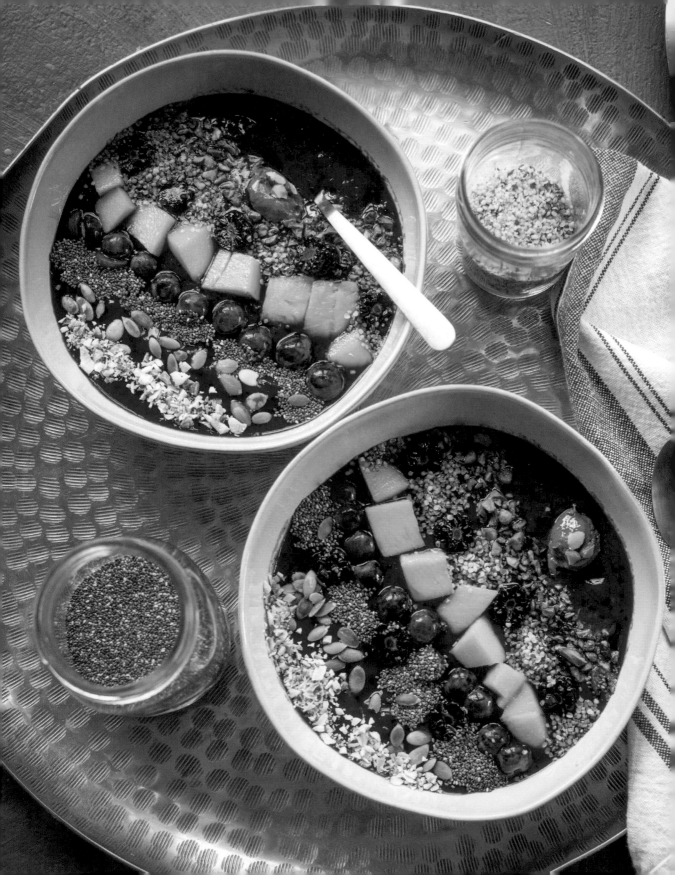

DRAGON FRUIT SMOOTHIE BOWL

Dragon fruit, also known as the strawberry pear, is one of the most beautiful fruits inside and out, and this colorful, exotic smoothie bowl is a breeze to make. The grapes, apple juice, and bananas deliver the sweetness, and the lemon gives the infusion of sassy tartness you need to slay the dragons in your life.

Yield: About 4 cups | *Serves 2 to 4*

One 12-ounce package frozen dragon fruit cubes (about 2 cups)

½ cup unsweetened apple juice

2 medium bananas, frozen

½ cup red seedless grapes

Juice of ¼ to ½ lemon, to taste

2 tablespoons almond or cashew butter

2 teaspoons maple syrup or honey

Toppings such as toasted coconut flakes, hemp hearts, chia seeds, chopped macadamia nuts, avocado, berries, sliced banana, cubed peaches, or granola

1. Combine the dragon fruit, apple juice, bananas, grapes, and lemon juice in a blender until smooth.

2. Divide the mixture into 4 bowls. Top each bowl with a tablespoon of nut butter and a swirl of maple syrup.

3. Add some fun and healthy toppings like hemp hearts and chia seeds.

PRO TIP: When bananas start to get a little past their prime, freeze them to use later in smoothies and smoothie bowls or in one of our frozen treat recipes (page 181).

CARROT CAKE PANCAKES
with Cashew Maple Syrup

I'm often asked by folks who juice a lot, "What do I do with all the pulp?" Our answer: Make these amazing pancakes. Our Carrot Cake Pancakes deliver the comfort-food feels of traditional pancakes but with the nutritional firepower of oats, flax, chia, cashew, cinnamon, allspice, and nutmeg. These will be a smash hit in your house!

Yield: 15 to 20 pancakes | *Serves 4*

2 tablespoons ground flaxseed

2 cups quick-cooking oats

1 ripe banana

1 teaspoon baking powder

1 tablespoon chia seeds

Juice of 1 lemon

1 teaspoon vanilla extract

½ teaspoon allspice

½ teaspoon cinnamon

⅛ teaspoon nutmeg

¼ teaspoon salt

2 cups unsweetened almond milk, plus more to thin batter as needed

1½ cups carrot pulp from your juicer or finely grated carrots

1 tablespoon coconut oil

Cashew Maple Syrup (recipe follows)

1. Combine the flaxseed and oats in a food processor until the oats are pulverized into a flour.

2. Add the banana, baking powder, chia seeds, lemon juice, vanilla, allspice, cinnamon, nutmeg, salt, and almond milk to the processor and blend until everything is well mixed.

3. Transfer the batter from the food processor to a large mixing bowl and combine it with the carrot pulp until the pulp is evenly distributed, ensuring that the batter has a thick yet pourable consistency. Thin the batter with almond milk as needed.

4. Heat a large pan over medium heat and brush the inside with coconut oil. In the warm pan, form the pancakes using about ⅛ cup of batter per pancake. Cook the pancakes for a few minutes per side, flipping them occasionally until each side is golden brown. Repeat until all the batter is used, making sure to brush the pan with coconut oil between batches if it looks dry.

5. Serve the pancakes warm with our Cashew Maple Syrup.

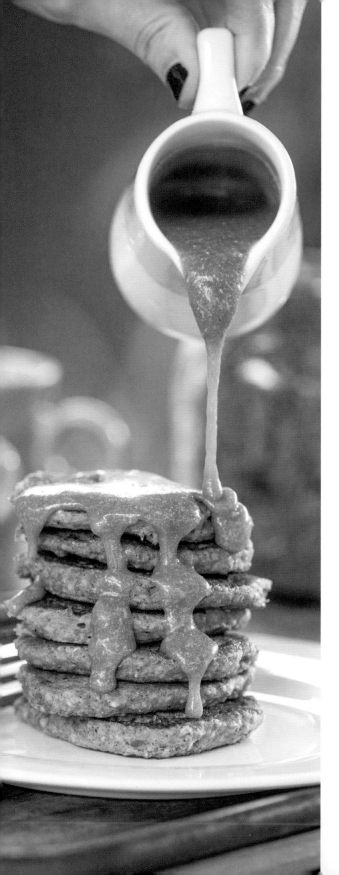

CASHEW MAPLE SYRUP

This two-ingredient sauce is far greater than the sum of its parts. One plus one equals ten!

¼ cup maple syrup
2 tablespoons cashew butter

1. Vigorously whisk the maple syrup and cashew butter in a small mixing bowl until smooth.

2. Warm and serve.

A study found that women who consumed the most nuts had 84 percent lower odds of breast cancer compared to those who consumed the least.[52]

CASHEW BUTTER TOAST

Looking for an ultra-fast, ultra-nutritious, ultra-tasty breakfast? Cashew butter toast is always a hit at our breakfast table. Feel free to substitute any nut butter of your choice. Micah likes cashew butter; I like almond butter. The topping options are endless.

Yield: 4 slices | *Serves 4*

4 slices sprouted whole-grain bread

¼ cup cashew butter

4 teaspoons hemp hearts

4 teaspoons chia seeds

Blueberries, blackberries, or raspberries, to taste

Sliced banana, fig, or strawberry, to taste

4 teaspoons honey or maple syrup

1. Toast the bread slices to a golden brown.

2. Spread the cashew butter onto each slice of toast, then sprinkle each with 1 teaspoon of hemp hearts and 1 teaspoon of chia seeds.

3. Top your toast with whatever fruit you like: blueberries, blackberries, raspberries, sliced bananas, figs, or strawberries, etc.

4. Drizzle with honey or maple syrup.

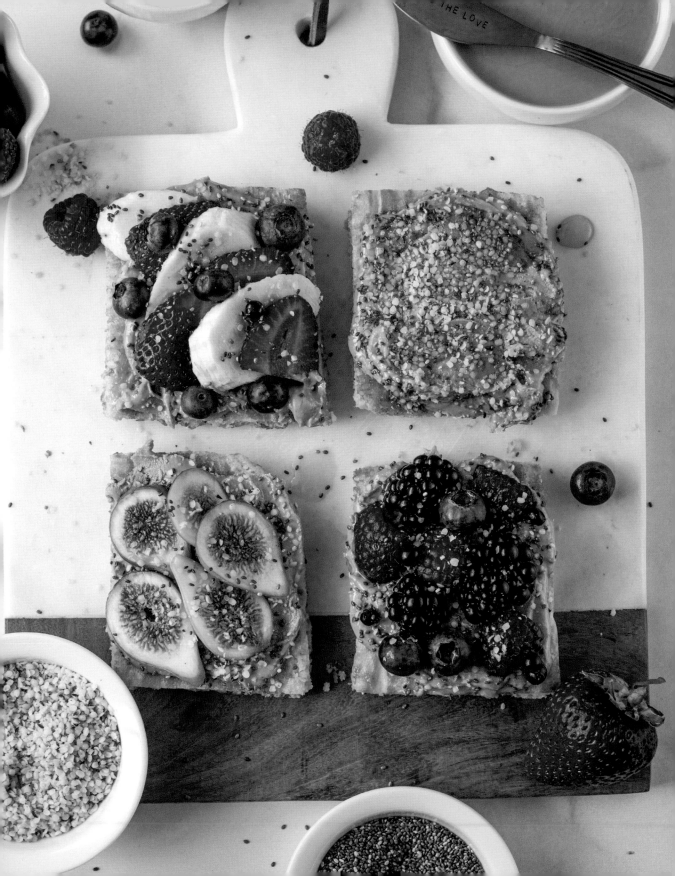

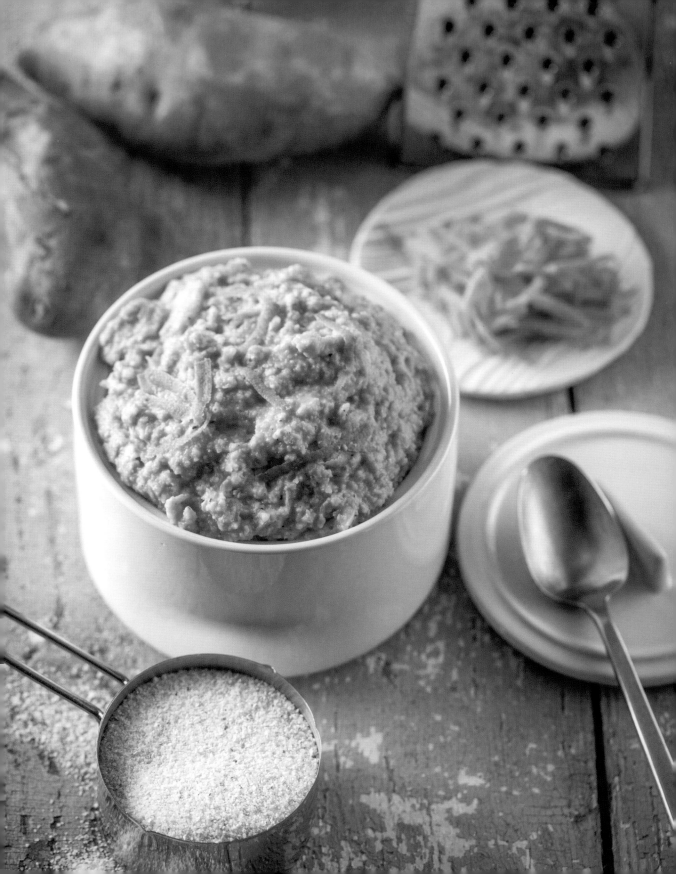

SWEET POTATO GRITS

This is our fun and tasty twist on traditional southern grits with amped-up nutritional value. Sweet potato adds a carotenoid-rich depth and sweetness, and the garlic and cayenne bring the spicy anticancer punch. Great for breakfast or as a savory dinner side. Our Sweet Potato Grits and BBQ Brussels Sprouts make a perfect pair.

Yield: About 5 cups | *Serves 4 to 6*

2 cups water

2 cups unsweetened almond milk

1 cup white or yellow corn grits*

1 medium sweet potato, peeled and grated (about 2 cups)

4 medium garlic cloves, peeled and smashed

¼ cup nutritional yeast

1 tablespoon apple cider vinegar

1 tablespoon extra-virgin olive oil

1 teaspoon black pepper

½ teaspoon sea salt

¼ teaspoon cayenne pepper (optional)

1. Combine the water and almond milk in a medium saucepan over high heat.

2. Slowly whisk in the grits as you bring the mixture up to a boil. This will prevent lumps.

3. Add the sweet potato, garlic, nutritional yeast, vinegar, olive oil, black pepper, salt, and cayenne pepper, if using, and stir to combine.

4. Reduce the heat to low, cover, and simmer for up to 30 minutes or according to the package instructions for the grits, stirring occasionally to keep from scorching.

*Most corn grown in the U.S. is genetically modified. To avoid this, buy organic corn grits.

Sweet potatoes provide one of the biggest nutritional bangs for your buck and contain a unique protein that has been found to slow down the growth, spread, and invasion of colorectal cancer cells.[53]

RED FLANNEL HASH

We whipped traditional corned beef hash into shape by swapping the beef for beets and pumped up the nutritional jams with sweet potato, paprika, coriander, and garlic. This is a fantastic side for breakfast, lunch, or dinner.

Yield: About 5 cups | *Serves 4*

1 medium red beet, peeled and diced (1 to 2 cups)

2 medium skin-on gold potatoes, diced (about 2 cups)

1 large skin-on sweet potato, diced (about 2 cups)

1 medium red onion, diced (about 1½ cups)

½ teaspoon paprika

½ teaspoon ground coriander

¼ teaspoon granulated garlic

½ teaspoon black pepper

½ teaspoon sea salt

2 tablespoons extra-virgin olive oil

1. Mix all the ingredients in a large cast-iron skillet or pan until well coated.

2. Spread the vegetables into a single layer and place the skillet in a cold oven.

3. Set your oven to 415°F and cook for 30 to 35 minutes or until all the vegetables are tender. Serve warm.

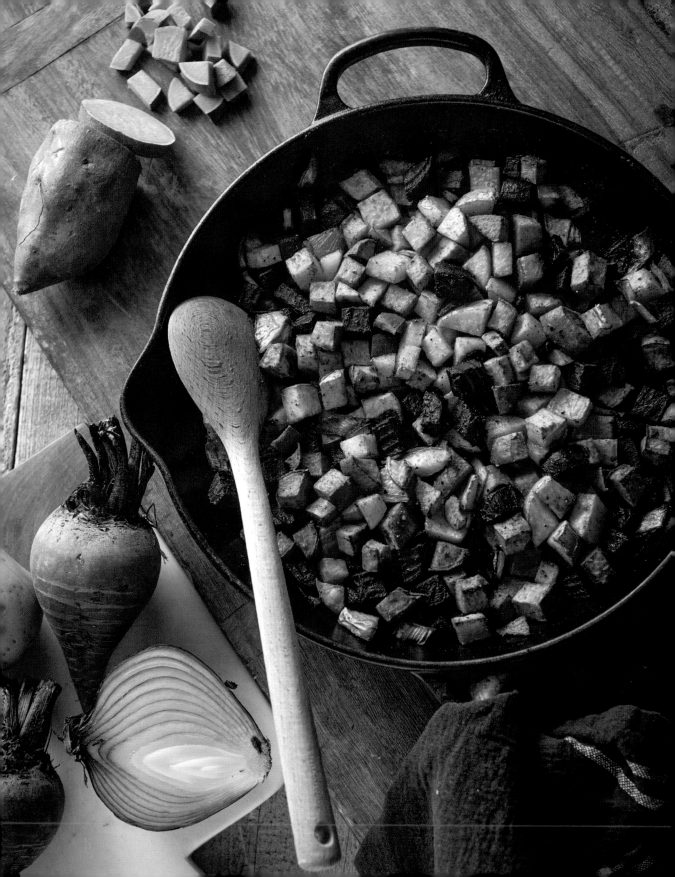

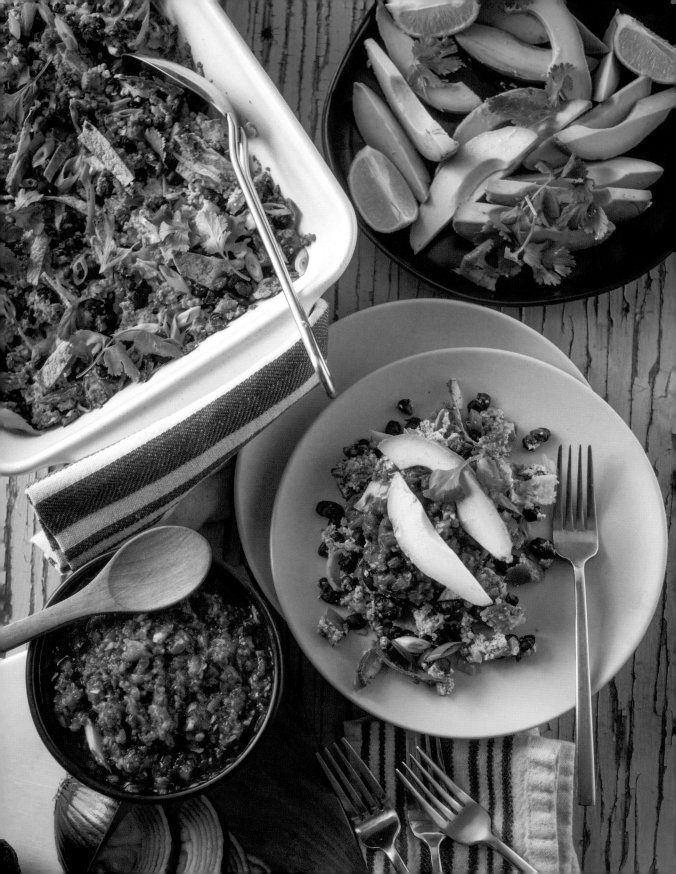

TOFU MIGAS BAKE

Migas means "crumbs" in Spanish and is a Tex-Mex breakfast dish typically served with left-over chips and scrambled eggs. Our plant-based version is quick and easy, super yummy, and loaded with anticancer goodness. Just toss the ingredients into a casserole dish, bake, and dig in. The guacamole on top really makes this dish, and the leftovers double as nachos.

Yield: 8 cups | *Serves 4 to 6*

One 14-ounce package extra-firm tofu, drained and crumbled

1 teaspoon cumin

1 teaspoon ground coriander

1 teaspoon turmeric

1/4 teaspoon granulated garlic

3/4 teaspoon sea salt

1/2 teaspoon black pepper

1 medium green bell pepper, diced

1/2 medium red onion, diced

One 15-ounce can black beans, drained and rinsed, or 1 1/2 cups cooked black beans

1 1/2 cups corn tortillas cut into strips (from about 4 to 5 taco-size tortillas)

2 tablespoons extra-virgin olive oil

2 cups guacamole or Guac of Ages (page 192)

Super-Fresh Salsa (optional, page 195)

Juicer Hot Sauce (optional, page 217)

1. Preheat your oven to 400°F.

2. Combine the tofu, cumin, coriander, turmeric, garlic, salt, black pepper, bell pepper, onion, beans, tortillas, and oil in a 9 x 12-inch casserole dish and mix well.

3. Using a spatula, lightly pack the mixture into an even layer and bake for 25 minutes.

4. Serve warm with a side of guacamole; top with salsa and hot sauce, if desired.

PRO TIP: Cooking tofu this way helps it absorb any sauces or spices you pair it with. Bake your tofu at the beginning of the week and have it at the ready for soups, salads, bowls, and stir-fries. You can jazz it up with our Spicy Nut Butter Sauce page 203 or Orange-Ginger Sauce page 119.

BREAKFAST BARS

Make a batch of these super-nutritious breakfast bars with oats, flax, chia, hemp, and your favorite nut butter and enjoy them all week. These also make great snacks for on-the-go, lunch boxes, or as an after-dinner treat. These stay in heavy rotation in our home.

Yield: 12 bars | *Serves 12*

1½ cups quick-cooking oats

1 cup coconut flakes, plus ¼ cup for the topping

1 cup golden raisins

¼ cup flaxseeds

¼ cup chia seeds

¼ cup hemp hearts

¼ teaspoon ground ginger

¼ teaspoon allspice

½ teaspoon cinnamon

¼ teaspoon sea salt

¼ cup maple syrup or honey

¾ cup smooth nut butter, such as almond, cashew, or peanut

1 teaspoon vanilla extract

1. Combine the oats, 1 cup of coconut flakes, raisins, flaxseeds, chia seeds, hemp hearts, ginger, allspice, cinnamon, and salt in a large mixing bowl.

2. Add the maple syrup or honey, nut butter, and vanilla extract to the mixing bowl. Knead the mixture with your hands until all ingredients are evenly mixed.

3. Press the mixture into the corners of a 9 x 9-inch baking pan lined with wax paper or parchment paper and pat it down evenly across the top.

4. Top with the remaining ¼ cup of coconut flakes, press them in, and chill the pan in the refrigerator for 1 hour.

5. Remove the pan and cut into rectangles. Store in the fridge in an airtight container to keep fresh, firm, and moist.

Hemp hearts are an incredible, nutritionally dense superfood. Three tablespoons of hemp hearts contain 10 grams of protein, 12 grams of omega-3 and omega-6 fats, and they are an excellent source of iron, phosphorus, magnesium, and manganese.

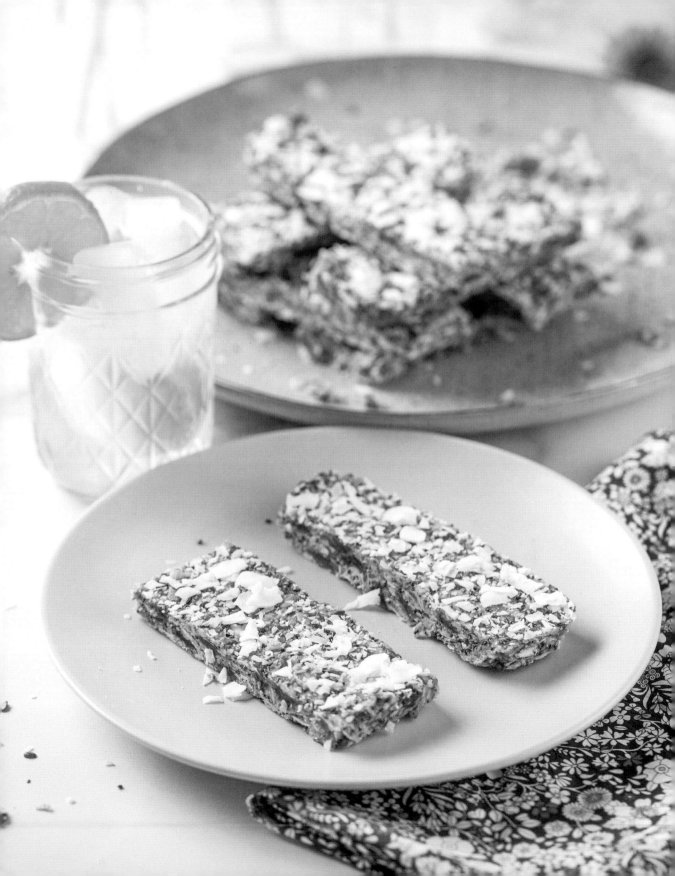

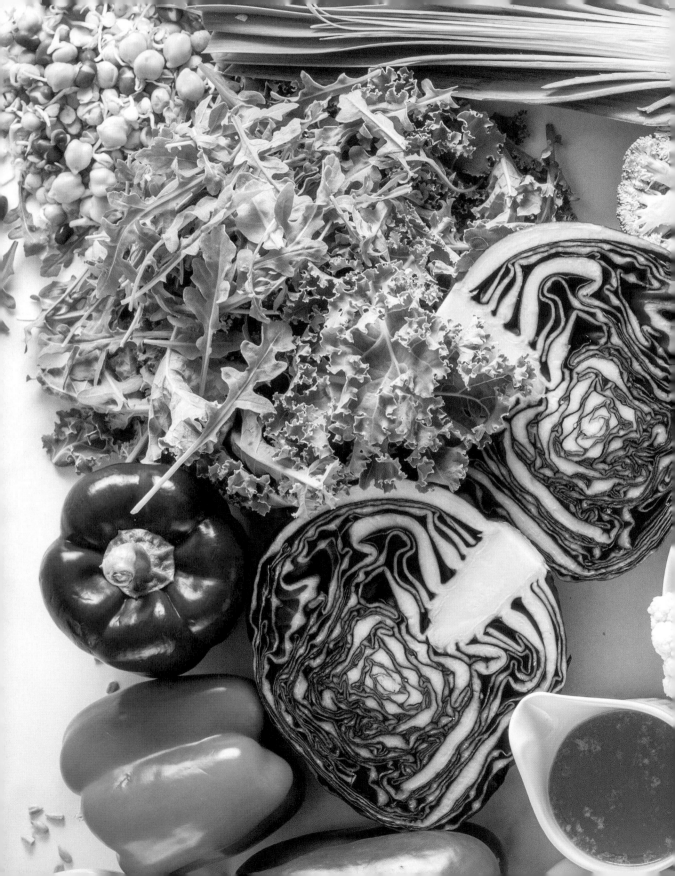

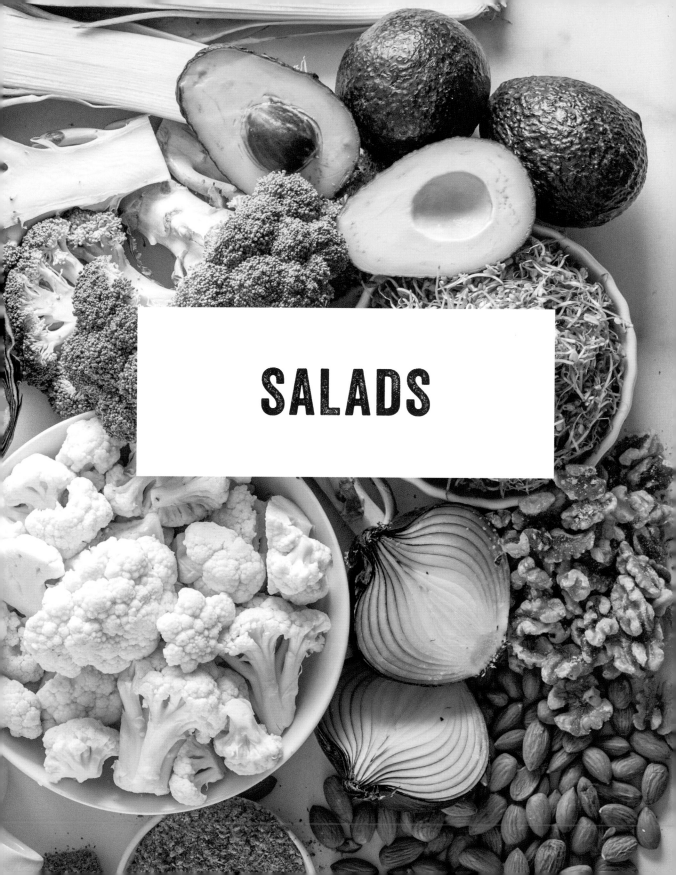

SALADS

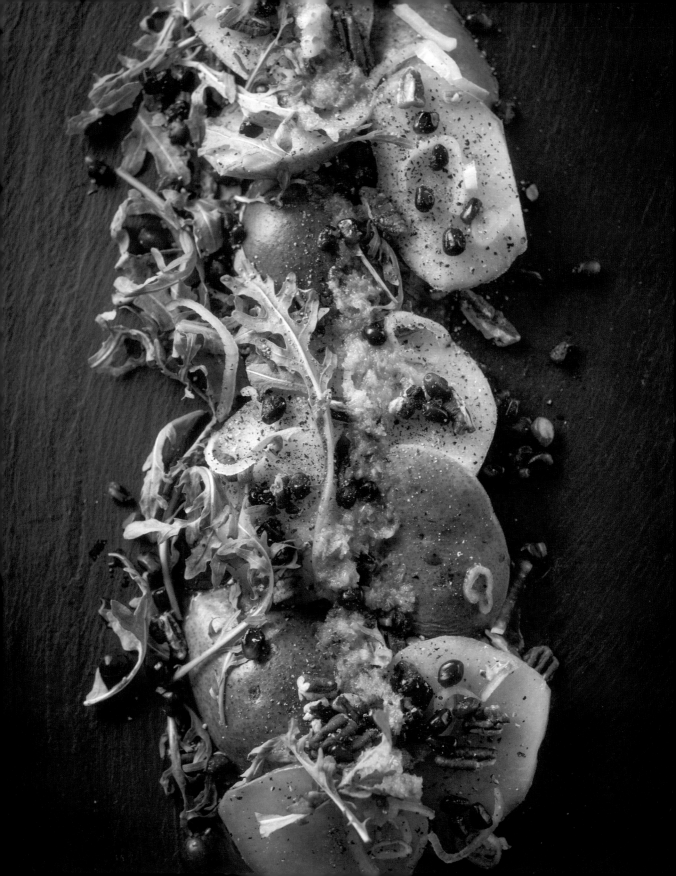

PEAR AND POMEGRANATE SALAD
with Maple Ginger Dressing

Hearty, sweet roasted pears, pomegranate seeds, toasted pecans, and Maple Ginger Dressing over a bed of spicy arugula. Are you drooling yet? This showstopping artisan salad will delight your taste buds.

Yield: 6 cups | *Serves 4 to 6*

Dressing

1 tablespoon fresh grated ginger

2 tablespoons maple syrup

1 tablespoon apple cider vinegar

1 tablespoon extra-virgin olive oil

¼ teaspoon sea salt

Salad

4 medium Anjou pears, cored and cut into thirds

Juice of 1 medium lemon

2 cups loose-packed baby arugula

½ cup toasted chopped pecans

¼ cup pomegranate seeds

1 medium shallot, thinly sliced

1. Preheat your oven to 350°F.

2. Combine the ginger, maple syrup, vinegar, olive oil, and salt in a medium Mason jar and shake until all the ingredients are mixed. Set aside.

3. Toss the pear slices in a medium bowl with lemon juice to prevent browning.

4. Place the pear slices on a parchment-lined baking sheet and bake for 15 minutes.

5. Transfer the warm pears to a large platter and garnish with arugula, pecans, pomegranate seeds, and shallot.

6. Drizzle with the Maple Ginger Dressing and serve.

SPICY WATERMELON AND PEPITA SALAD

This is our take on a popular Mexican street snack in which fresh fruit is dusted with spicy dried pepper and lime. We paired fresh watermelon with a dressing of jalapeño, onion, lime, maple syrup, and pumpkin seeds. This sweet and spicy summer snack is so good you may be tempted to keep it all for yourself.

Makes 16 slices | *Serves 4 to 6*

Dressing

1 tablespoon extra-virgin olive oil

2 tablespoons maple syrup

Juice of 2 medium limes

Salad

1 small seedless watermelon, sliced into triangles

½ small red onion, sliced

1 large jalapeño pepper, thinly sliced

⅓ cup roasted salted pepitas

Sea salt and black pepper, to taste

1. Whisk the olive oil, maple syrup, and lime juice in a medium bowl and set aside.

2. Shingle the watermelon slices on a large rimmed platter and garnish with the onion and jalapeño.

3. Drizzle the dressing evenly over the salad and garnish with the pepitas, salt, and pepper.

PRO TIP: Control the spiciness by removing the seeds and slicing the jalapeño super thin. You can also serve the jalapeños on the side.

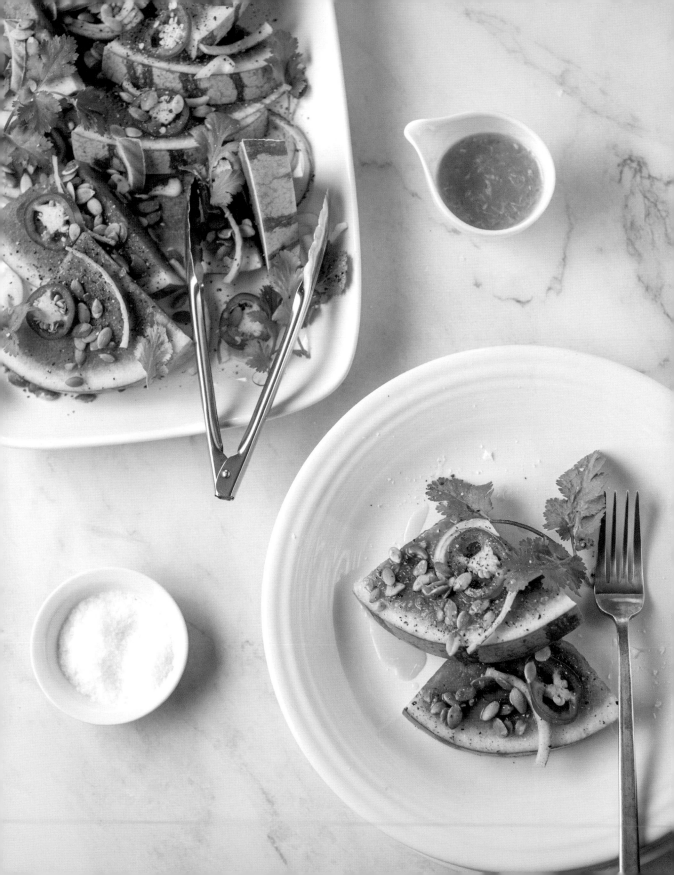

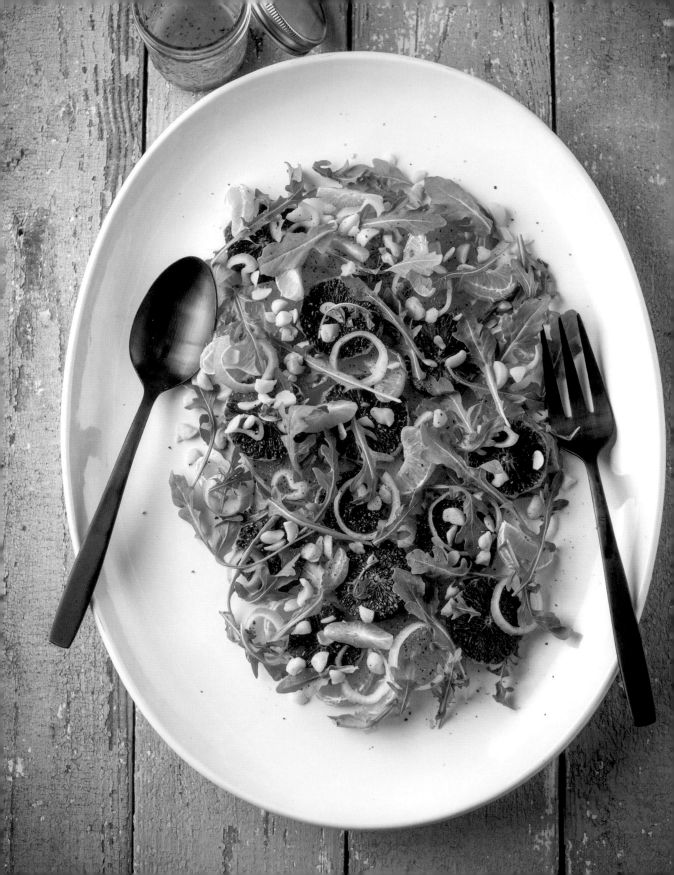

BLOOD ORANGE AND MACADAMIA NUT SALAD

This punchy, wonderful dish takes oranges out of the snack bowl and onto the dinner table, putting the citrus center stage. Blood oranges are not only beautiful but are also a perfect balance of sweetness and acidity. The peppery arugula and hearty macadamia nuts give you an über-delicious summer salad that will bring the house down.

Yield: 6 to 8 cups | *Serves 4*

Dressing

2 teaspoons extra-virgin olive oil

2 teaspoons maple syrup

¼ teaspoon black pepper

Juice of 1 lemon

Salad

1 large navel orange, peeled and sliced

3 medium blood oranges, peeled and sliced

2 clementines or tangerines, peeled and pulled into segments

1 medium shallot, sliced and rinsed with water

1½ cups baby arugula

¼ cup chopped macadamia nuts

1. Add the olive oil, maple syrup, pepper, and lemon juice to a small Mason jar, screw on the lid, and shake to combine. Set aside.

2. Lay out the navel oranges, blood oranges, and clementines in an overlapping pattern on a large platter, punctuating the larger shapes with the clementine pieces.

3. Top the citrus with the shallot, arugula, and macadamia nuts, and drizzle the dressing over the top.

PRO TIP: Blood orange season is from late winter to spring. If you are unable to find blood oranges or you just want to switch it up a bit, use 2 small grapefruits instead.

CASHEW CAESAR SALAD
with Roasted Chickpeas

Our mouthwatering lemony cashew Caesar dressing over a bed of crunchy romaine with roasted chickpeas and sweet apple will delight any Caesar salad lover, even the emperor himself!

Yield: 8 cups | *Serves 4*

1½ cups cooked chickpeas or one 15-ounce can chickpeas, drained and rinsed

1 tablespoon extra-virgin olive oil

½ teaspoon garlic powder

½ teaspoon chili powder

Salt, to taste

Zest and juice of 1 medium lemon

1 tablespoon grainy mustard

2 tablespoons cashew butter

1 teaspoon liquid aminos

1 tablespoon tamari

1 tablespoon maple syrup

¼ cup plus 2 tablespoons nutritional yeast, divided

¼ teaspoon crushed red pepper (optional)

Black pepper, to taste

1 to 2 heads romaine lettuce, chopped into 1-inch pieces

1 apple, diced (use your favorite sweet variety)

1. Preheat your oven to 400°F.

2. Combine the chickpeas, olive oil, garlic powder, and chili powder with a few pinches of salt in a medium bowl and toss to coat.

3. Spread the chickpeas into a single layer on a parchment-lined baking sheet and bake for 30 to 40 minutes, until the chickpeas are crispy.

4. Combine the lemon zest and juice, mustard, cashew butter, liquid aminos, maple syrup, ¼ cup nutritional yeast, red pepper, and black pepper in a large bowl and whisk until smooth. Add water 1 tablespoon at a time until a pourable consistency is reached.

5. Add the romaine to the bowl and toss to coat.

6. Add the baked chickpeas and apples to the top of the salad mixture and garnish with the remaining 2 tablespoons of nutritional yeast.

NOTE: For a savory version, substitute quartered artichoke hearts for the apples and bake them with the chickpeas.

PRO TIP: Wrap this salad in a sprouted whole-grain tortilla for a healthy and complete meal on the go. It's a lunch-box favorite around here!

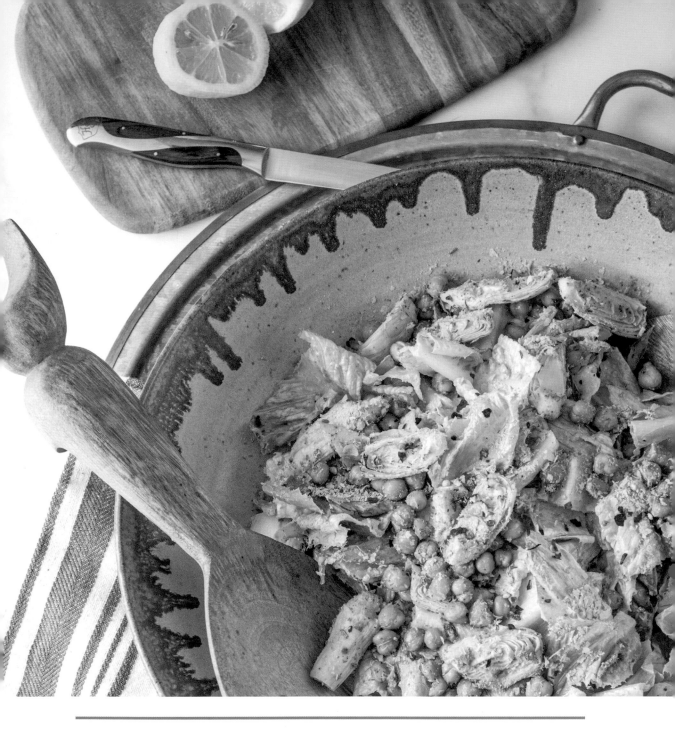

Apples contain unique anticancer polyphenols and flavonoids like quercetin. Eating an apple per day could decrease your risk of colorectal cancer by 35 percent. Eating more than one apple per day could reduce your risk by 50 percent![54]

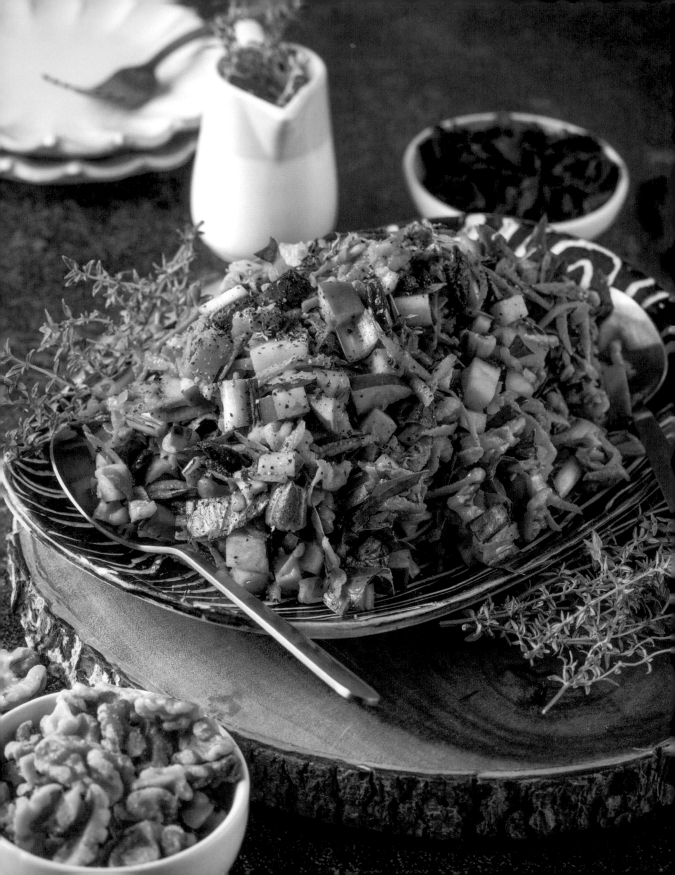

DANDELION APPLE GOJI SALAD

Dandelion greens are an incredibly nutritious and potent anticancer food but are rarely consumed because most folks don't know they are edible, and they are slightly bitter. We cracked the code and created a beautiful flavor balance by adding sweet apples, goji berries, and a maple mustard dressing. This superfood salad has a wide spectrum of flavors and textures and a hearty, satisfying crunch.

Yield: 6 cups | *Serves 4 to 6*

Dressing

Juice of 1 lemon

1 tablespoon extra-virgin olive oil

2 tablespoons maple syrup

2 tablespoons grainy mustard

1 tablespoon minced shallot

¼ teaspoon sea salt

¼ teaspoon black pepper

Salad

1 medium Pink Lady or other sweet apple, diced (about 1½ cups)

4 medium carrots, shredded (about 2 cups)

1 medium bunch dandelion greens, chopped (about 2 cups)

½ cup chopped walnuts

½ cup dried goji berries

1 teaspoon fresh thyme leaves

1. Whisk all the ingredients for the dressing in a large bowl until well incorporated.

2. Add all the ingredients for the salad to the bowl with the dressing and toss to combine.

PRO TIP: This salad can be made and stored in the fridge for up to 3 days and enjoyed as a quick lunch or side with dinner.

Dandelion greens are a super-nutritious source of vitamins A, K, C, and B_6, thiamin, riboflavin, calcium, iron, potassium, manganese, folate, magnesium, phosphorus, and copper.

AVOCADO CAPRESE SALAD

Our plant-based take on the classic Italian caprese salad is one of Micah's favorite quick dishes. We love to use fresh tomatoes and basil from the garden with sliced avocado instead of mozzarella. This salad is refreshing and perfect for a summer lunch.

Serves 4 to 6

2 medium avocados, sliced

2 medium tomatoes, sliced

About 12 fresh basil leaves

2 tablespoons balsamic vinegar

2 tablespoons pine nuts

Black pepper and sea salt, to taste

1. Shingle alternating slices of avocado and tomato on a large platter until all the slices are used.

2. Tuck the basil leaves between the slices of avocado and tomato.

3. Pour the balsamic vinegar onto the plate and allow it to season the salad from the under-side. This makes for a neater presentation.

4. Garnish the salad with pine nuts, black pepper, and sea salt.

PRO TIP: To expand the flavor, toast the pine nuts. Preheat your oven to 350°F. Arrange the pine nuts in a single layer on a small sheet pan. Toast them for 5 minutes, or until fragrant.

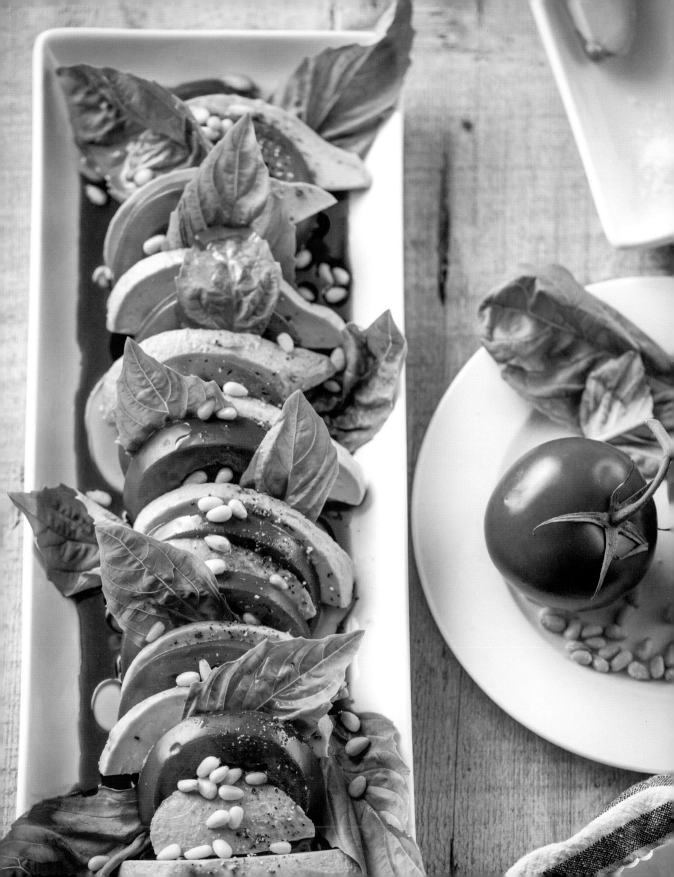

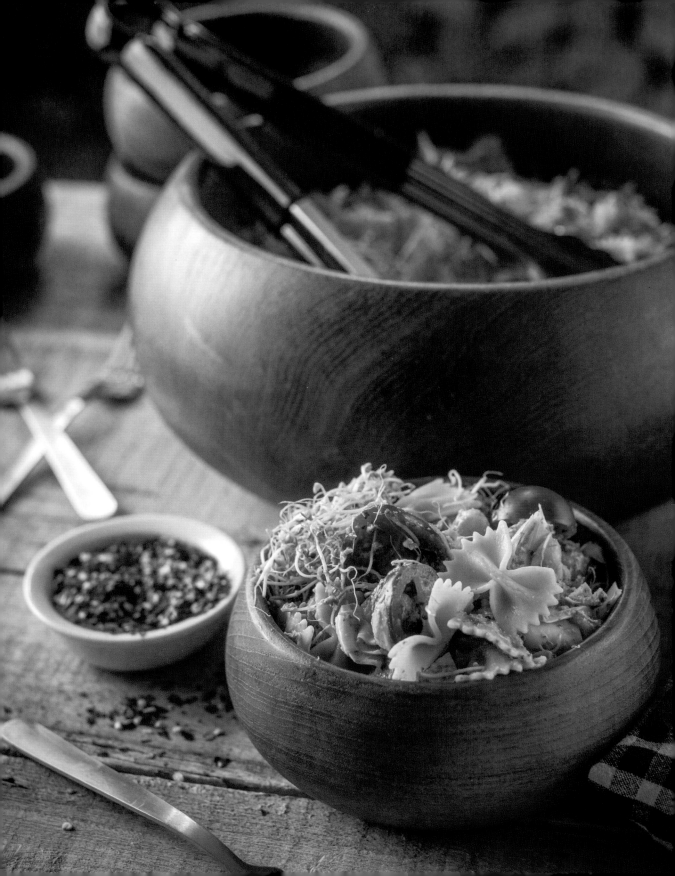

BROCCOLI SPROUT PESTO PASTA SALAD

This pasta salad is next level! It delivers all the happy belly feels of traditional pasta salad, but with the added anticancer kick of our peppery broccoli sprout pesto. Perfect for the lunch box, picnic basket, or potluck.

Yield: 8 cups | *Serves 4*

½ pound chickpea or lentil pasta, such as farfalle or rotini

1½ cups Broccoli Sprout Pesto (page 188)

One 14-ounce can artichoke hearts, drained and roughly chopped

1 pint cherry tomatoes, halved

2 medium celery ribs, thinly sliced

One 15-ounce can chickpeas, drained

1 teaspoon crushed red pepper

1. Cook the pasta according to the package instructions, rinse under cold water, and drain.

2. Toss the Broccoli Sprout Pesto (page 188) with the cooled and drained pasta in a large bowl along with the remaining ingredients until everything is coated in pesto.

ETHIOPIAN-STYLE BEET AND LENTIL SALAD

I absolutely adore Ethiopian cuisine. This dish combines many of the flavors of a traditional Ethiopian vegetable platter all into one salad. The unique combination of rosemary, jalapeño, and garlic adds serious wow factor.

Yield: 6 cups | *Serves 4 to 6*

3 medium beets

1 teaspoon minced ginger

½ teaspoon minced garlic

½ teaspoon minced rosemary

Juice of 1 lemon

1 tablespoon extra-virgin olive oil

¼ teaspoon sea salt

1 pint cherry tomatoes, halved

1 cup sprouted or cooked lentils

1 small jalapeño, sliced

2 cups arugula

1. Preheat your oven to 350°F.

2. Wrap the beets in parchment paper and place on a baking sheet. Bake for 1 hour. Allow the beets to cool enough to handle.

3. Scrub the beets with a paper towel to remove the skin. Discard the skin.

4. Dice the beets, discarding the top roots.

5. Toss the beets, ginger, garlic, rosemary, lemon juice, olive oil, salt, tomatoes, lentils, and jalapeño together in a large mixing bowl.

6. Place the arugula in a serving bowl or on a platter and top with the beet and lentil mixture.

PRO TIP: If you buy beets with the greens still attached, you can use the greens just like any other green leafy veggie. They're delicious sautéed with some onion and a little olive oil or tossed into a smoothie or salad. Just make sure to clean the beet greens thoroughly to remove the dirt.

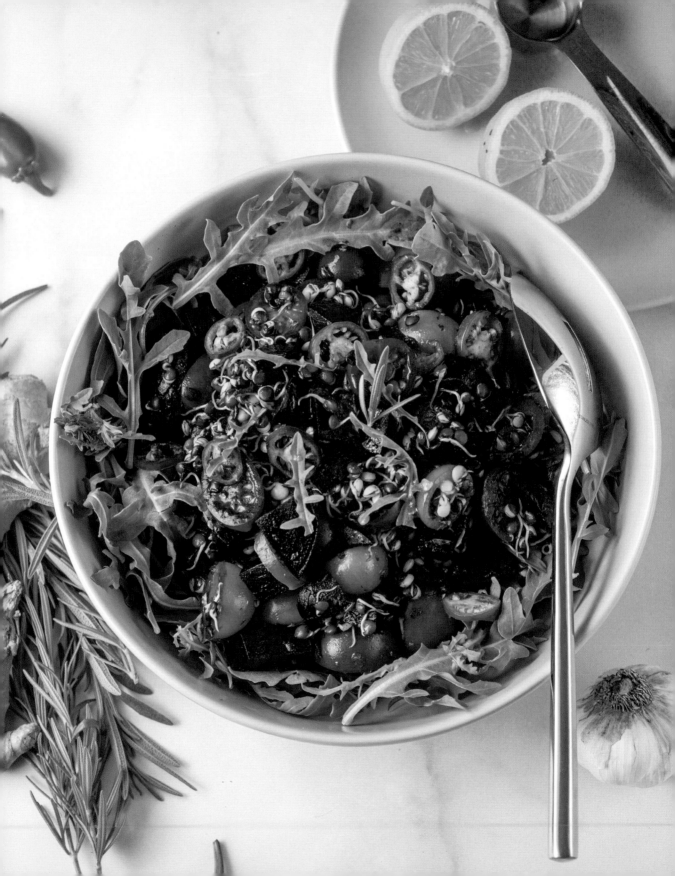

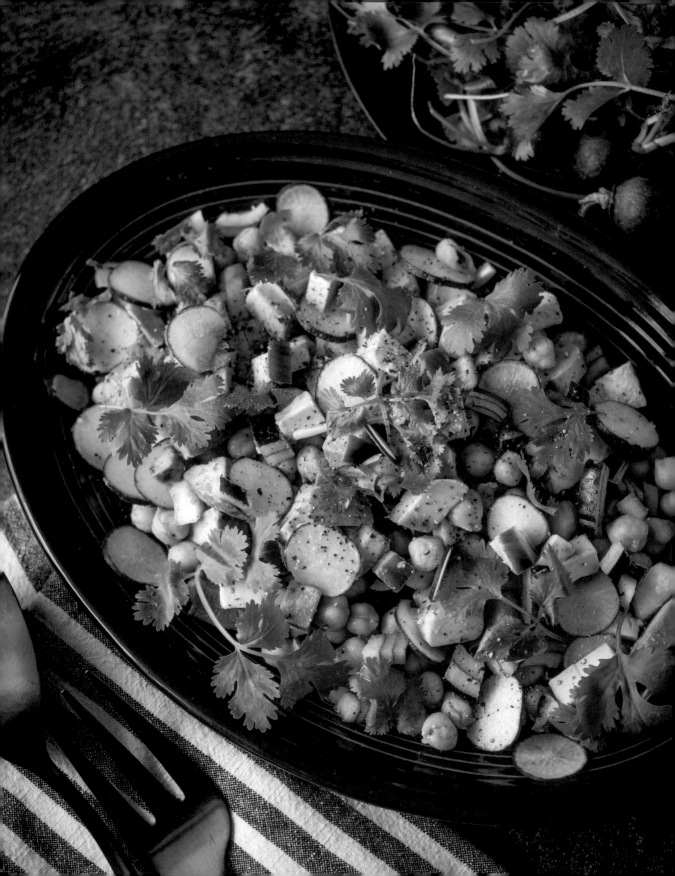

GARBANZO BEAN AND AVOCADO SALAD

This is a quick and easy salad that Micah often makes for lunch. It's light but keeps you satisfied until dinnertime. The lime and cilantro are bright and refreshing, and the radishes and red onion really make it pop. This is super yummy.

Yield: 4 cups | *Serves 4*

One 15-ounce can chickpeas, drained, or 1 ½ cups cooked chickpeas*

½ medium red onion, diced (about 1 cup)

⅔ cup sliced radish

½ teaspoon ground coriander

¼ teaspoon sea salt

1 to 3 tablespoons flax oil or olive oil

Juice of 1 lime

1 medium avocado, diced

½ cup cilantro, to garnish

1. Place all the ingredients except the cilantro in a large mixing bowl and toss to combine.

2. Serve the salad on a platter or on individual dishes garnished with fresh cilantro.

PRO TIP: To jazz up this recipe, feel free to add more raw veggies like broccoli, cauliflower, and sweet peppers.

*Pinto beans are a good substitute for chickpeas.

A study found that women who consumed the most legumes (chickpeas, lentils, peas, and beans) had 46 percent lower odds of breast cancer than those who consumed the least.[55]

BAKED FALAFEL SALAD WRAPS
with Maple Tahini Dressing

Falafel is a popular Middle Eastern street food made from chickpeas (or fava beans), fresh herbs, and spices that are formed into small patties and fried. Our falafel is baked, not fried, and served in lettuce wraps instead of pita bread, topped with our scrumptious Maple Tahini Dressing. It's a little messy and a lot yummy.

Yield: 4 wraps | *Serves 4*

1 cup dried chickpeas, soaked overnight and drained

1 cup loose-packed parsley, plus more for garnish

1 cup loose-packed cilantro

Juice and zest of 1 large lemon

1 teaspoon ground coriander

1 teaspoon cumin

1 teaspoon sea salt

4 garlic cloves

2 tablespoons garbanzo bean (chickpea) flour

½ teaspoon baking powder

1 serrano pepper (optional)

2 tablespoons extra-virgin olive oil, divided

1 medium head romaine or green leaf lettuce

Maple Tahini Dressing (recipe follows)

1 small cucumber, sliced

2 medium Roma tomatoes, diced

½ small yellow or white onion, thinly sliced

1. Preheat your oven to 425°F.

2. Blend the chickpeas, parsley, cilantro, lemon juice and zest, ground coriander, cumin, salt, garlic, garbanzo bean flour, baking powder, and serrano pepper, if using, in the work bowl of your food processor until a coarse green dough is formed. Set aside in the fridge for 20 minutes.

3. Brush 1 tablespoon of olive oil on a parchment-lined sheet pan.

4. With lightly wet hands, form 1 tablespoon of the falafel dough into a ball and flatten it slightly on the sheet pan. Repeat until all the dough is used. You should get about 20 falafels.

5. Brush the tops of the flattened falafel balls with the remaining tablespoon of olive oil and bake for 20 minutes.

6. Make the Maple Tahini Dressing and set aside in the fridge until you're ready to eat.

7. Remove the falafel from your oven and stuff 4 or 5 into a stack of 3 large lettuce leaves.

8. Garnish with the Maple Tahini Dressing, cucumber, tomato, onion, and parsley. Repeat the process to make 4 wraps.

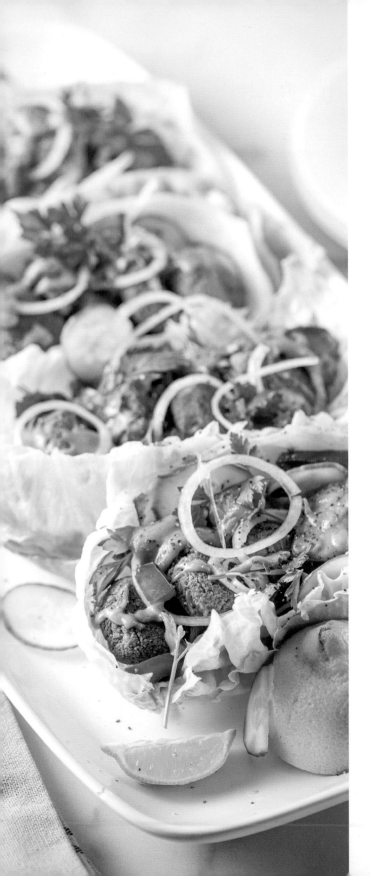

MAPLE TAHINI DRESSING

Yield: About ½ cup | *Serves 4*

¼ cup tahini
2 tablespoons maple syrup
Juice of 1 medium lemon

1. Whisk all the ingredients together in a medium bowl until smooth.

2. Set aside in the fridge until ready to use.

NOTE: If the dressing is too thick, add a little water to thin it out.

NOTE: This recipe does not work with canned chickpeas. We've tried! So plan to soak your dried chickpeas for 8 hours or overnight for the best, freshest falafel you'll ever have.

PRO TIP: Feel free to use sprouted whole-grain pita bread instead of lettuce wraps if you like!

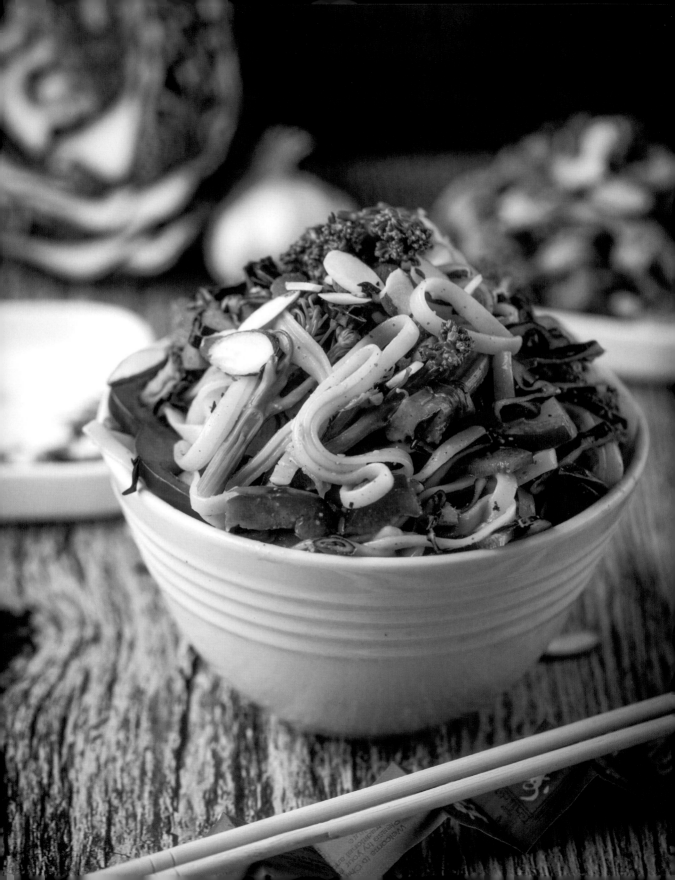

BROCCOLI NOODLE SALAD

This Asian-inspired noodle salad with anticancer superstars broccolini, purple cabbage, and green onions and topped with our Spicy Nut Butter Sauce will delight your soul and your senses.

Yield: 8 cups | *Serves 4 to 6*

Dressing

Spicy Nut Butter Sauce (page 203)

Salad

One 8-ounce package pad thai rice noodles

1 large bunch broccolini, chopped, about 3 cups

2 cups thinly sliced purple cabbage

1 bunch green onions, chopped

1 red bell pepper, sliced

¼ cup sliced almonds, toasted

1. Whisk in an additional ½ cup of water into the Spicy Nut Butter Sauce.

2. Cook the noodles according to the package directions. Remove the noodles from the pot, saving the hot water in the pot, and cool the noodles under running water.

3. Bring the pot of water back to a boil, blanch the broccolini for about 30 seconds, and then cool under running water.

4. Place the noodles and broccolini in a large mixing bowl. Add the thinned Spicy Nut Butter Sauce, cabbage, onions, and bell pepper and toss to combine.

5. Garnish the salad with almonds and serve chilled or at room temperature.

PRO TIP: Look for brown, red, or black pad thai rice noodles for a nutritional boost. Find them in the international section of your grocery store or online.

CHARLENE'S MASON JAR SUMMER SALAD

Our photographer Justin's grandmother Charlene loved to make this salad in the summer and fall when tomatoes, cucumbers, and onions were in season. This delicious salad is perfect for a light lunch or as a side with cooked veggies, like our Southern Veggie Plate (page 122). It's also a "quick pickle," a way to preserve some of your summer produce and enjoy it later in the week.

Yield: 4 cups | *Serves 4*

1 cup water

½ cup apple cider vinegar

½ teaspoon sea salt

2 teaspoons maple syrup

1 ½ heaping cups sliced tomatoes

1 ½ heaping cups sliced cucumbers

1 cup sliced onion

1 medium jalapeño, sliced lengthwise

Garden herbs, black pepper, and olive oil, to garnish

Special equipment:

1 quart-size Mason jar

1. Place the water, vinegar, salt, and maple syrup in a quart-size Mason jar. Screw on the lid and shake the jar until the salt and maple syrup dissolve.

2. Layer the tomatoes, cucumbers, onions, and jalapeño into the jar.

3. Refrigerate for at least an hour or up to a week before serving.

4. To serve, remove the tomatoes, cucumber, and onions from the jar, top with fresh herbs like thyme and parsley, and garnish with black pepper and a light drizzle of olive oil.

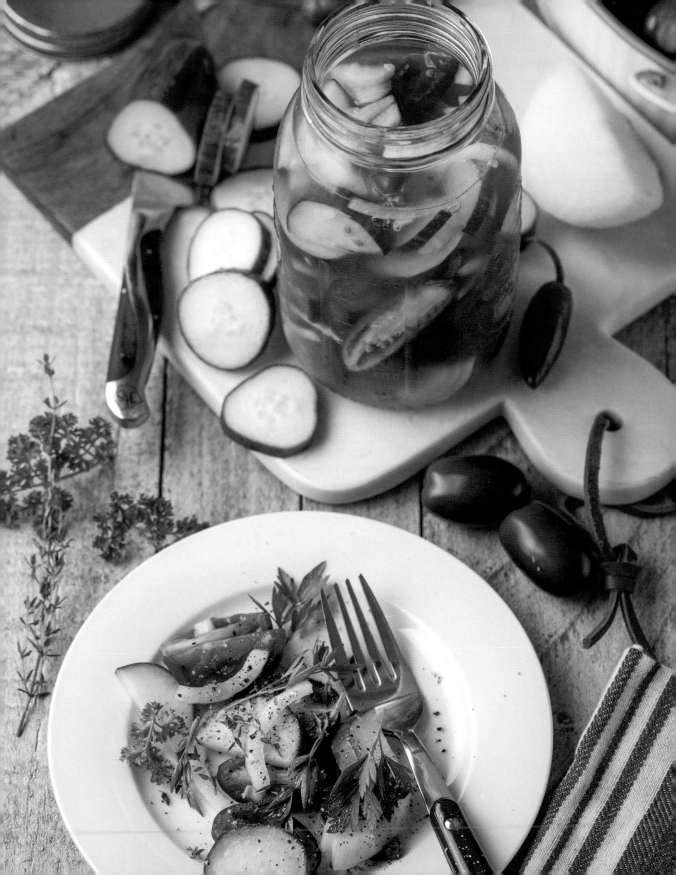

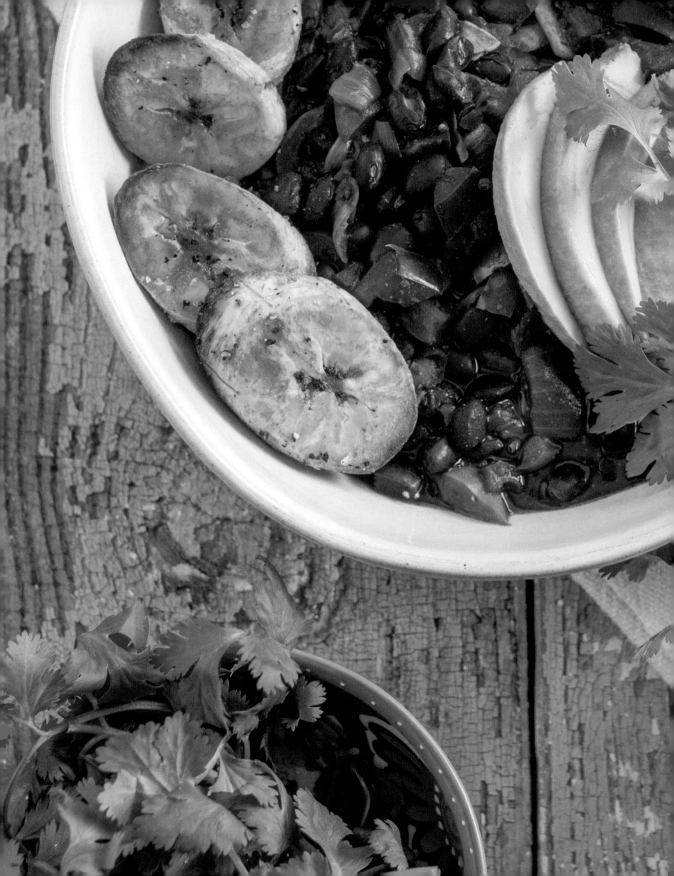

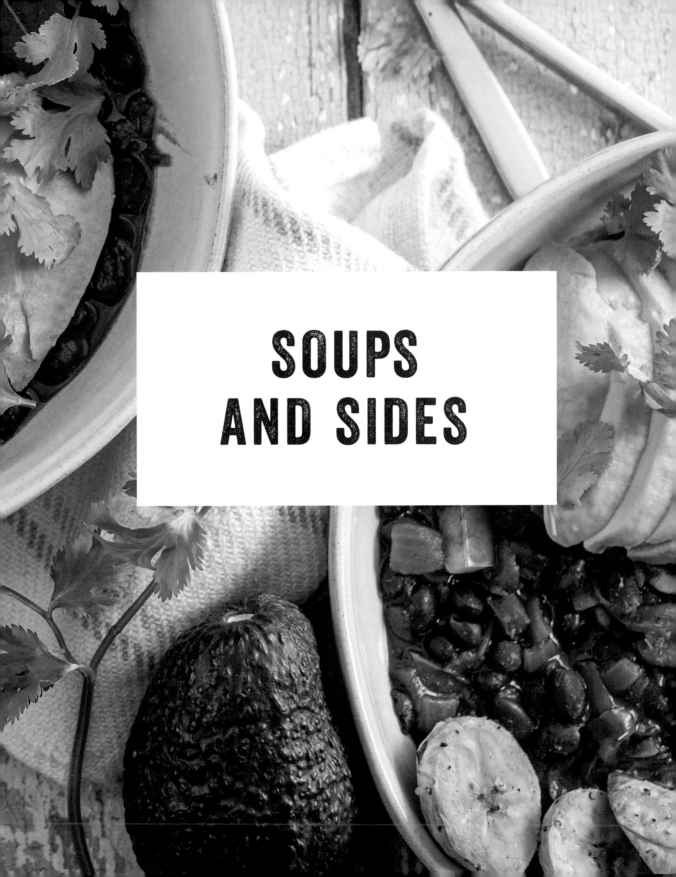

SOUPS
AND SIDES

INDIAN STEW

Our Indian Stew is a delightful blend of sweetness, spice, and savory flavors. Wait until you taste the cherries! This dish is on heavy rotation in our kitchen in the fall and winter months, and I could easily eat it every day for the rest of my life.

Yield: 14 cups | *Serves 6 to 8*

4 cups brown rice

1 medium onion, chopped

8 garlic cloves, peeled

2-inch piece of fresh ginger

2 tablespoons curry powder

1 teaspoon ground coriander

1 teaspoon cumin

½ teaspoon cinnamon

1 tablespoon maple syrup

1 tablespoon apple cider vinegar

2 tablespoons coconut aminos*

1 medium jalapeño (optional)

1 tablespoon extra-virgin olive oil

½ cup dry lentils

One 28-ounce can crushed tomatoes

3 cups unsweetened almond milk

1 cup chopped unsweetened dried cherries, divided

1 large russet potato, diced, 3 cups (peeling optional)

1 medium bell pepper, diced, 1¼ cup

1 medium head of cauliflower, broken into florets, 5 to 6 cups

4 medium carrots, diced, 2 cups

1 cup frozen green peas

1 cup cashews

½ cup cilantro leaves

PRO TIP: Dried cherries add a nice pop of sweetness to this deeply spiced curry. You can also use golden raisins or currants.

*If you can't get coconut aminos, use 1 tablespoon of tamari, a low-sodium soy sauce.

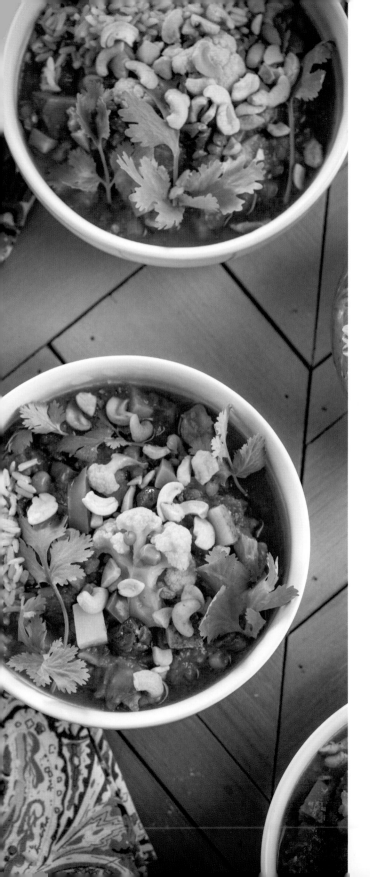

1. Make the rice according to the package directions and keep warm until ready to serve.

2. Combine the onion, garlic, ginger, curry powder, coriander, cumin, cinnamon, maple syrup, vinegar, coconut aminos, and jalapeño, if using, in a food processor until a paste forms and all ingredients are thoroughly blended.

3. Set a large soup pot or Dutch oven over medium-high heat and add the olive oil and blended curry paste. Cook, stirring frequently, until most of the moisture has evaporated and the paste becomes very thick.

4. Add the lentils, tomatoes, and milk. Stir, cover, and allow the mixture to cook for 10 minutes to soften the lentils.

5. Add ¹/₂ cup of the cherries to the pot, along with the potato, pepper, cauliflower, carrots, and peas. Cover and reduce the heat to a simmer. Cook for 25 minutes or until the vegetables are tender.

6. Serve the stew over brown rice and garnish with the remaining ¹/₂ cup of cherries, plus the cashews and cilantro leaves.

COLLARD AND CASHEW SWEET POTATO TAGINE

Tagine is a North African stew traditionally made in an earthenware pot. Our version with lemon and apricots is unbelievably good. This dish never fails to deliver cozy comfort-food vibes, and I get so excited every time Micah tells me she's making it for dinner.

Yield: 8 cups | *Serves 4 to 6*

1 tablespoon extra-virgin olive oil

1 medium onion, diced

8 garlic cloves, minced

1 tablespoon minced ginger

1 medium serrano pepper, minced

4 cups vegetable broth

2 cups water

6 ounces tomato paste

½ cup cashew butter

1 medium skin-on sweet potato, diced

1 tablespoon harissa*

One 15-ounce can chickpeas, drained, or 1½ cups cooked chickpeas

1 medium lemon, quartered

½ cup diced dried apricots

½ to 1 bunch collard greens, ribs removed and leaves finely chopped**

½ teaspoon salt

½ cup chopped cashews

Cilantro, to garnish

Super Sriracha, to garnish (page 210)

1. Sauté the oil, onion, garlic, ginger, and serrano pepper in a Dutch oven or tagine over medium-high heat for 5 minutes, or until the onion is translucent.

2. Add the vegetable broth, water, tomato paste, and cashew butter, bring to a gentle boil, then stir vigorously to mix the tomato paste and cashew butter evenly. Add the sweet potato, harissa, chickpeas, lemon, apricots, collard greens, and salt.

3. Bring the mixture to a simmer, turn the heat down to low, and cover. Cook for 30 minutes, or until the sweet potatoes are tender, stirring occasionally.

4. Serve warm, topped with cashews and garnished with cilantro and a drizzle of sriracha.

*Harissa is a Moroccan spice mixture typically consisting of garlic, cumin, paprika, and coriander.

**Kale can be substituted for collard greens.

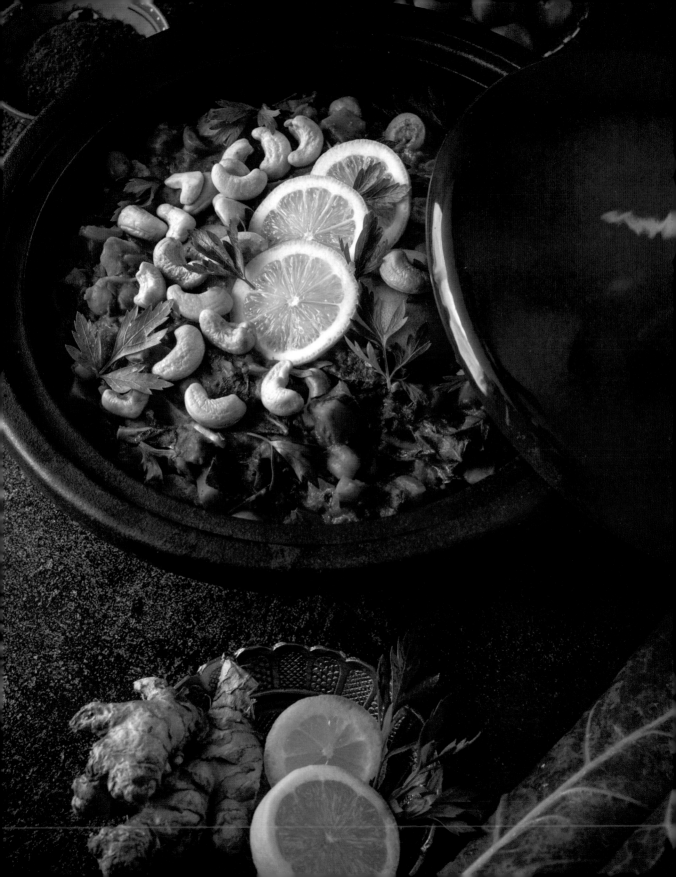

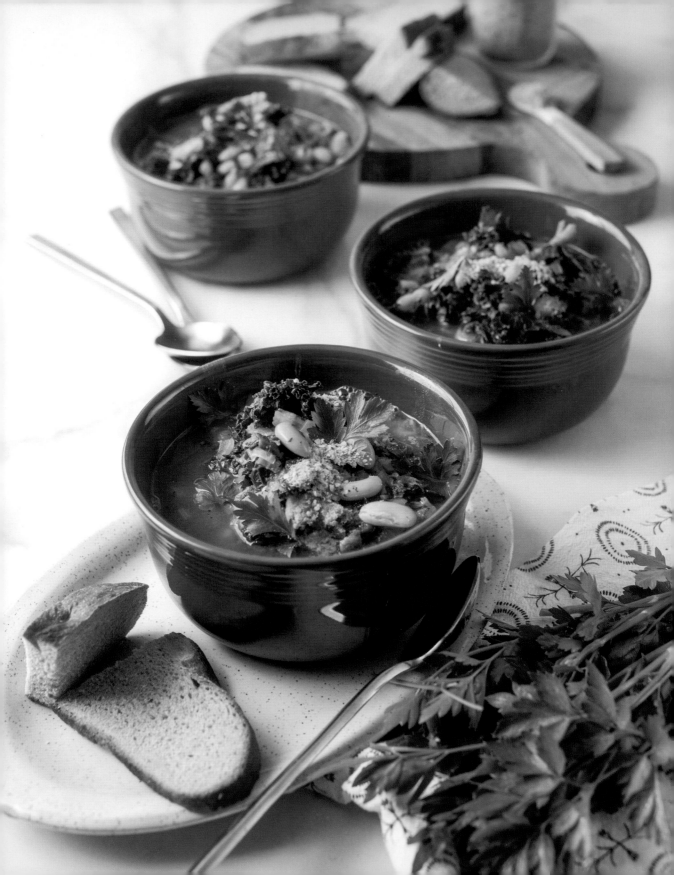

KALE AND WHITE BEAN SOUP

Soups are a great way to get super-nutritious greens like kale into your body. This hearty Tuscan staple with immune-boosting beans, mushrooms, garlic, and onions really hits the spot on a chilly day.

Yield: 8 cups | *Serves 6*

1 tablespoon extra-virgin olive oil

1 medium white onion, diced

2 celery ribs, diced

6 large garlic cloves, minced

One 8-ounce package whole baby bella or cremini mushrooms, smashed

1 bunch curly kale, stems removed and leafy parts roughly chopped

Two 15-ounce cans cannellini beans with liquid, or 3 cups cooked beans with 1½ cups water

Zest and juice of 2 lemons

1 tablespoon Italian seasoning or Bragg Organic Sprinkle

3 cups vegetable broth or Juicer Broth (page 214)

No Harm Parm (page 196), to garnish

1. Sauté the olive oil and onion in a large stockpot over medium-high heat for 5 minutes, or until the onion is translucent.

2. Add the celery, garlic, mushrooms, kale, beans with their liquid, lemon zest and juice, Italian seasoning, and broth and bring to a boil.

3. Reduce the heat to a simmer, cover, and cook for 20 minutes.

4. Garnish with No Harm Parm (page 196) and serve warm.

NOTE: Instead of slicing the mushrooms, use the palm of your hand and smash them flat. This is a rustic, fun way to add hearty texture to a meat-free stew.

Mushrooms and Green Tea vs. Breast Cancer

The rate of breast cancer in American women is six times higher than in Asian women. Two protective dietary factors that have been identified are green tea and mushrooms. A 2009 study found that Chinese women who ate an average of only 15 mushrooms per month along with drinking 15 cups of green tea per month had an astounding 90 percent reduced risk of developing breast cancer when compared to women who didn't consume green tea or mushrooms regularly.[56]

TEMPEH BLACK BEAN CHILI

Crumbled tempeh plays the part of ground beef in this weeknight-ready dish. With just the right amount of spice and the perfect texture, this is a chili that the whole family will enjoy.

Yield: 8 cups | *Serves 4 to 6*

1 to 2 tablespoons extra-virgin olive oil

1 large red onion, diced

1 red bell pepper, diced

1 medium jalapeño, seeded and minced

4 garlic cloves, minced

1 tablespoon chili powder

1 teaspoon paprika

1 tablespoon cumin

½ teaspoon ground coriander

½ teaspoon sea salt

One 28-ounce can diced tomatoes with liquid

Two 15-ounce cans black beans, drained and rinsed, or 3 cups cooked beans

One 15-ounce can kidney beans, drained and rinsed, or 1½ cups cooked beans

One 8-ounce package tempeh, crumbled

2 tablespoons apple cider vinegar

1 bay leaf

2 cups water

1 teaspoon maple syrup

1 cup cilantro leaves

1 cup sliced green onion

2 avocados, sliced

1 lime, sliced

NOTE: Tempeh is made from whole soybeans, fermented and pressed into a firm cake so that it can be sliced, crumbled, or cubed. It has a much hardier texture than tofu.

1. Place the olive oil, onion, bell pepper, jalapeño, and garlic in a large pot over medium-high heat and cook, stirring often, for about 10 minutes, or until the onion starts to brown.

2. Add the chili powder, paprika, cumin, coriander, sea salt, tomatoes with liquid, beans, tempeh, vinegar, bay leaf, water, and maple syrup and stir to combine.

3. Reduce the heat to a simmer and cook, covered, for 25 minutes. Then uncover and cook for an additional 10 minutes.

4. Garnish with cilantro, green onion, avocado slices, and a squeeze of lime.

RECIPE VARIATION: At Step 2, instead of tempeh, add 1¼ cups of cooked black lentils with ½ cup of finely chopped walnuts. (A ½ cup of dried lentils yields roughly 1¼ cups cooked.)

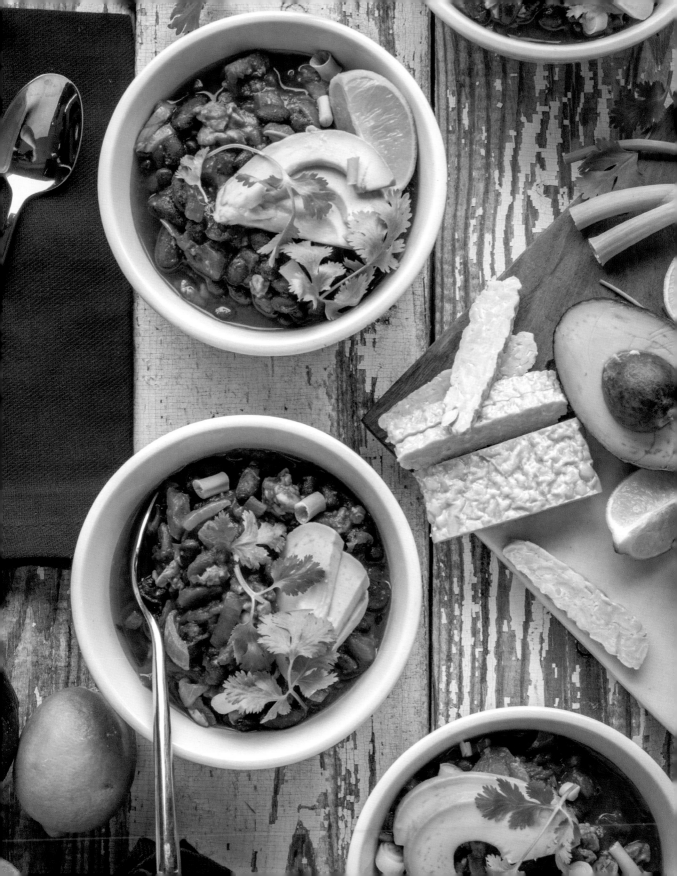

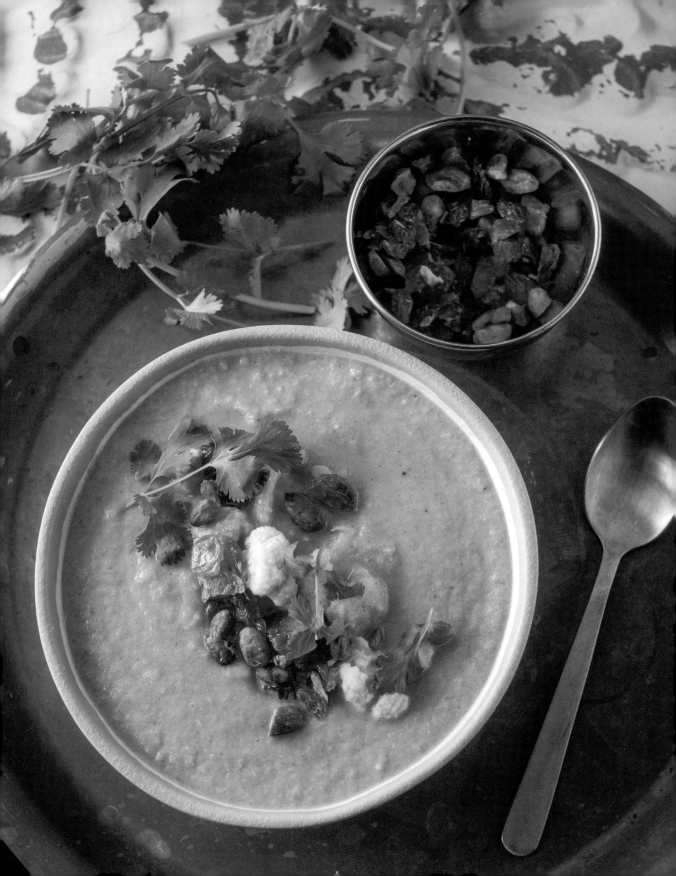

CURRIED CAULIFLOWER SOUP

We adore Indian and Thai cuisines, especially curries, and this cauliflower soup with creamy coconut milk, spicy jalapeños, and sweet golden raisins is just perfect.

Yield: 10 cups | *Serves 6*

1 tablespoon extra-virgin olive oil

1 tablespoon curry powder

1 teaspoon ground coriander

1 tablespoon chopped fresh ginger

8 medium garlic cloves, minced

1 medium white onion, chopped

1 medium Roma tomato, chopped

1 medium jalapeño, chopped

1 large cauliflower, florets and stems separated, roughly chopped (about 6 cups)

Zest and juice of 1 lime

One 13.5-ounce can coconut milk

2 cups vegetable broth or Juicer Broth (page 214)

Pistachios or cashews and golden raisins, to garnish

Salt, to taste

1. Add the oil, curry powder, and coriander to a large pot and heat at medium-high.

2. Once the oil starts to bubble and the curry becomes fragrant, add the ginger, garlic, onion, tomato, and jalapeño and cook for 8 minutes, or until the onion is translucent, stirring frequently.

3. Add the cauliflower stems, lime zest and juice, coconut milk, and broth.

4. Cover and simmer for 20 minutes, or until the cauliflower is tender.

5. Blend the soup with a hand mixer or in a blender until smooth, then return it to the pot.

6. Add the cauliflower florets and cook 10 minutes, or until just tender.

7. Ladle the soup into bowls and garnish with nuts, golden raisins, and a pinch of salt to taste.

ROASTED RAINBOW CARROTS EN PAPILLOTE

with Peanut and Carrot Top Pesto

En papillote means "in paper," which is a way to keep the moisture and flavor in during cooking. And the pesto is made with the carrot tops. This is a plant-based "nose-to-tail" recipe. No waste and unbelievably delicious!

Yield: 10 to 12 medium carrots | *Serves 4*

1 pound rainbow carrots with tops, ends trimmed, and carrots tops reserved

2 cups loose-packed carrot tops

½ cup peanuts

2 garlic cloves

Juice of 1 lemon

1 teaspoon maple syrup

2 tablespoons apple cider vinegar

1 tablespoon extra-virgin olive oil

1 tablespoon water

¼ teaspoon sea salt

¼ teaspoon black pepper

1. Preheat your oven to 400°F.

2. To wrap carrots *en papillote*, first tear off a sheet of parchment paper 3 times as long as the longest carrot.

3. Place the carrots lengthwise on the parchment.

4. Fold the parchment over the carrots. Then fold the open ends to create a pouch and crease the paper so that it stays folded. (It doesn't need to be airtight. We just want the moisture to stay inside the pouch as the carrots cook.)

5. Bake the carrots for 40 minutes.

6. Blend the remaining ingredients in the work bowl of your food processor until well mixed.

7. Using kitchen shears, carefully cut open the carrot papillote, taking extra care not to let the steam get you.

8. Slather the carrots with the pesto and enjoy.

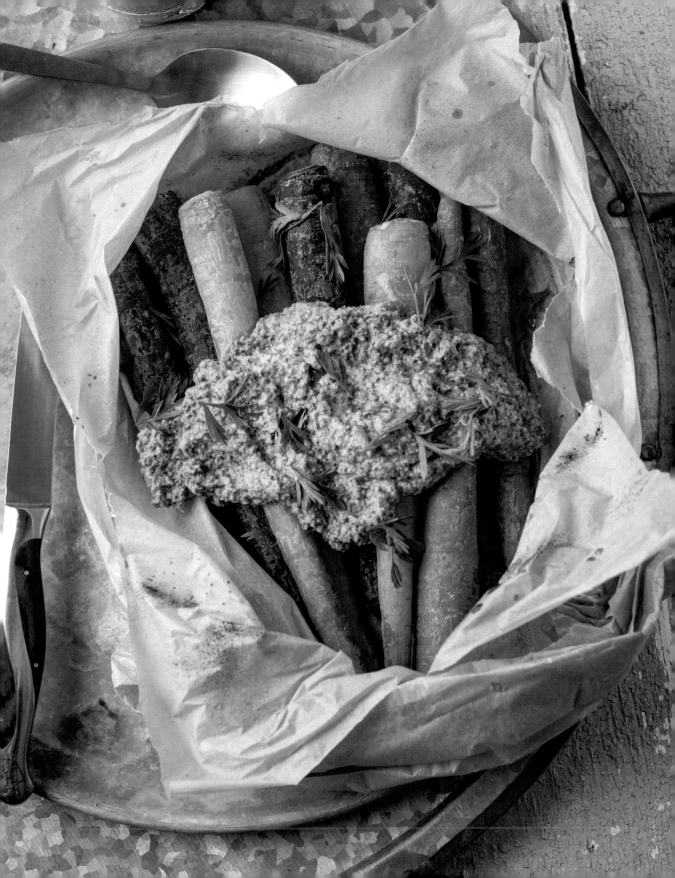

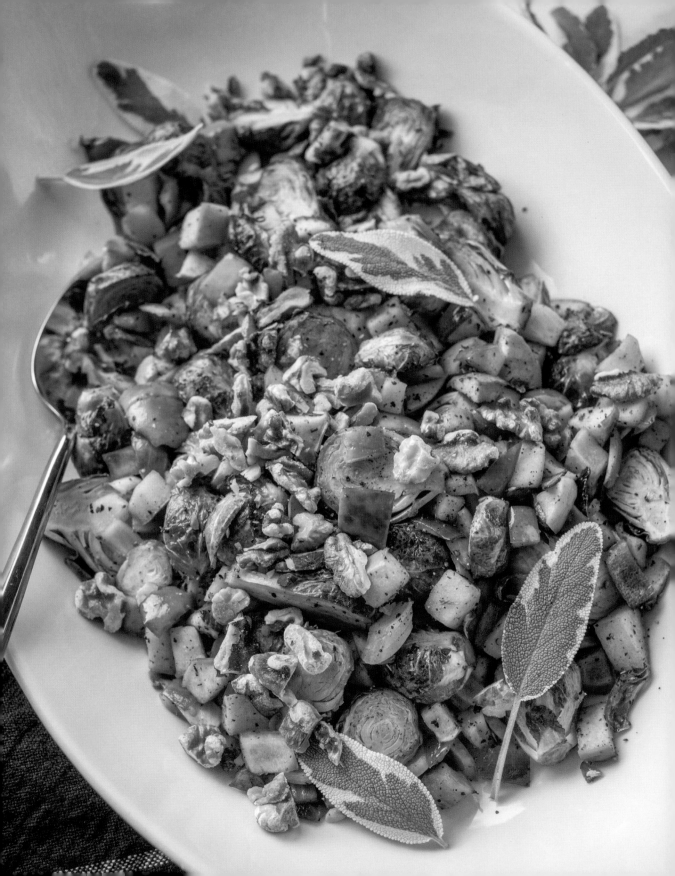

MAPLE BRUSSELS SPROUTS
with Sweet Apples

A touch of sweetness from apples and maple syrup takes Brussels sprouts over the rainbow. This is a great way to reintroduce cruciferous anticancer Brussels sprouts to anyone who isn't a fan. The first bite is like that magical moment when *The Wizard of Oz* goes from black and white to color. It's perfect for potlucks or holiday gatherings.

Yield: 5 cups | *Serves 4 to 6*

2 tablespoons apple cider vinegar

1 pound Brussels sprouts, halved

2 Fuji, Gala, Pink Lady, or other sweet apples, diced (about 2 cups)

1 small purple onion, diced (about 1½ cups)

1 tablespoon maple syrup

1 tablespoon toasted sesame oil

½ teaspoon sea salt

½ teaspoon black pepper

½ teaspoon dried sage

½ cup chopped walnuts

1. Preheat your oven to 350°F.

2. Combine all the ingredients except the walnuts in a large mixing bowl.

3. Spread the mixture out flat on a large, parchment-lined baking sheet.

4. Bake for 30 minutes, adding the walnuts for the last 5 minutes to toast. Serve warm.

One apple contains about 100 million bacteria, roughly 90 percent of which is found in the core and seeds, which is why I always eat the core and seeds. A study in Austria found that organic apples had a much more diverse population of bacteria than conventionally grown apples and contained the beneficial bacteria *Lactobacillus*, which was absent in conventional apples.[57]

MEXICAN STREET CORN
with Avocado Mayo

This is our tasty twist on traditional Mexican street corn. It always hits the spot and is the perfect complement to any rice and beans dish. Substituting avocado for mayonnaise makes this even more delicious and nutritious.

Yield: 5 cups | *Serves 5 to 6*

1 cup loosely packed cilantro leaves, plus additional for garnish

Juice of 2 medium limes

Zest of 1 medium lime

½ teaspoon cumin

½ teaspoon ground coriander

½ teaspoon salt

½ teaspoon black pepper

2 medium avocados, pitted and peeled

1 tablespoon extra-virgin olive oil

4 ears fresh corn, peeled, cooked, and kernels cut, or 4 cups frozen corn, cooked

1 large jalapeño, minced

3 green onions, sliced, tops reserved for garnish

1. To make the Avocado Mayo: Blend the cilantro, lime juice and zest, cumin, coriander, salt, pepper, avocados, and olive oil in the work bowl of your food processor until very smooth.

2. Toss the corn, jalapeño, and onions with the Avocado Mayo in a medium bowl. Garnish with sliced green onion tops and cilantro.

3. Serve warm or cold.

PRO TIP: Make a batch of our creamy Avocado Mayo to go on top of sandwiches, salads, and potatoes. It's delish!

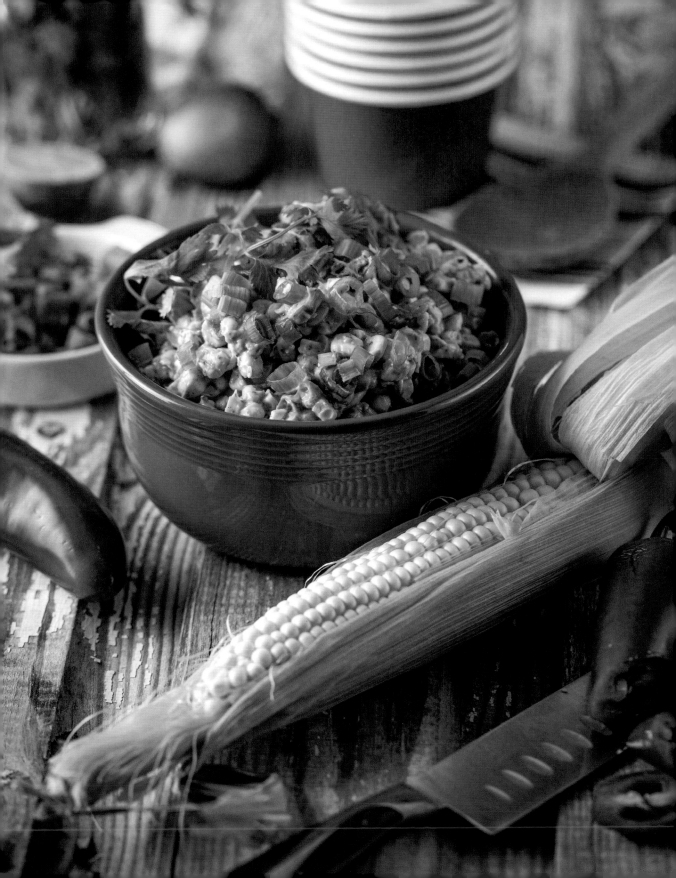

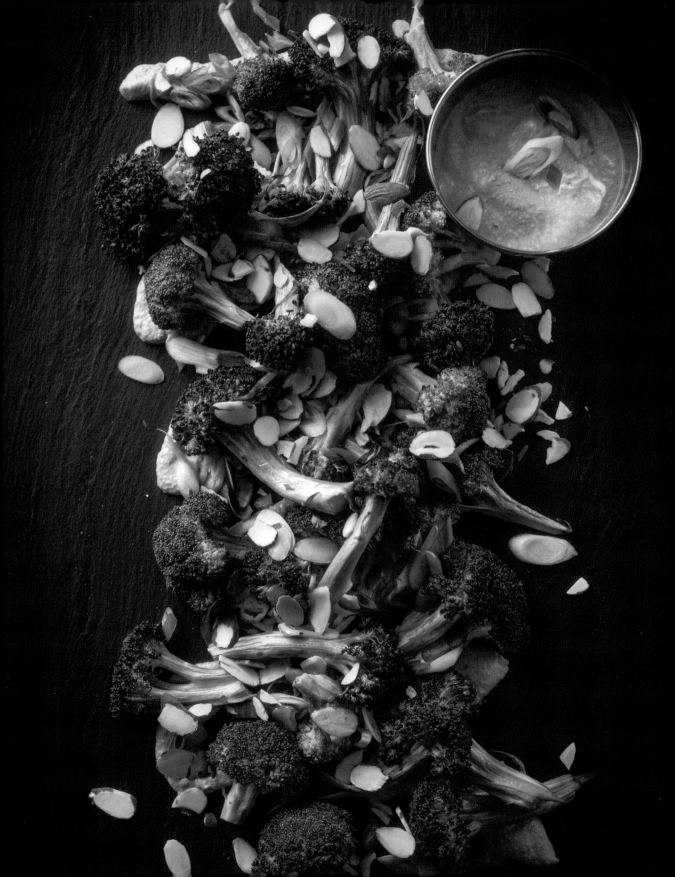

KIMCHI CASHEW BROCCOLI

Cruciferous cousins, broccoli and cabbage are powerful immune-boosting anticancer foods, and this sophisticated side will delight your taste buds. This dish is amazing, amazing, amazing, amazing.

Yield: 6 cups | *Serves 4*

6 to 7 cups broccoli (from about 1 large head)

1 teaspoon toasted sesame oil

1 tablespoon rice vinegar or apple cider vinegar

1 tablespoon coconut aminos

1 cup kimchi with liquid

1 cup raw cashews

Juice of 1 lime

1 teaspoon sriracha (optional)

¼ to ½ cup water

¼ cup sliced almonds, toasted

1. Toss together the broccoli, sesame oil, vinegar, and coconut aminos in a large mixing bowl until the broccoli is well coated.

2. Spread the broccoli in a single layer on a parchment-lined baking sheet and place the baking sheet into a cold oven.

3. Turn on your oven to 350°F and cook for 20 to 25 minutes. (This method cooks the broccoli all the way through without burning the edges too much.)

4. Blend the kimchi with its liquid, the cashews, lime juice, water, and sriracha, if using, in the work bowl of a food processor until smooth.

5. Spoon ½ of the Kimchi Cashew sauce onto 4 plates and top with the roasted broccoli and sliced almonds. Serve extra sauce on the side or reserve for another use.

PRO TIP: You can also skip the roasting and serve as a cold broccoli salad.

Sesame seeds and sesame oil contain an anticancer compound called sesamin, which has been shown to inhibit the proliferation of a wide variety of tumor cells, including leukemia, multiple myeloma, and cancers of the colon, prostate, breast, pancreas, and lung.[58]

QUINOA TABBOULEH

You need more parsley in your life, and tabbouleh, which is the most delicious parsley dish on the planet, is the way to do it. Our version of this Mediterranean staple uses the super seed quinoa instead of couscous. This quick and refreshing recipe is perfect as a light lunch or tasty side.

Yield: 4 cups | *Serves 4*

3 cups quinoa, cooked and cooled

2 tablespoons extra-virgin olive oil

1 teaspoon maple syrup

4 medium Roma tomatoes, diced

1 medium shallot, minced

1 medium garlic clove, minced

Zest and juice of 1 large lemon

½ teaspoon sea salt

1 bunch parsley, chopped

¼ cup chopped mint

1. Combine all the ingredients in a large mixing bowl.

2. Refrigerate until ready to serve.

PRO TIP: Rinse the finely diced shallot under cold water in a mesh strainer to reduce the astringent taste that raw onion can develop as the onion juice oxidizes.

Parsley contains the anticancer compound apigenin. Apigenin blocks aromatase, an enzyme in the body that helps promote the cancer-promoting hormone estrogen and inhibits breast and prostate cancer cells.[59] Apigenin has also been found to make cancer cells more sensitive to chemotherapy by activating a tumor-suppressor gene called p53.[60]

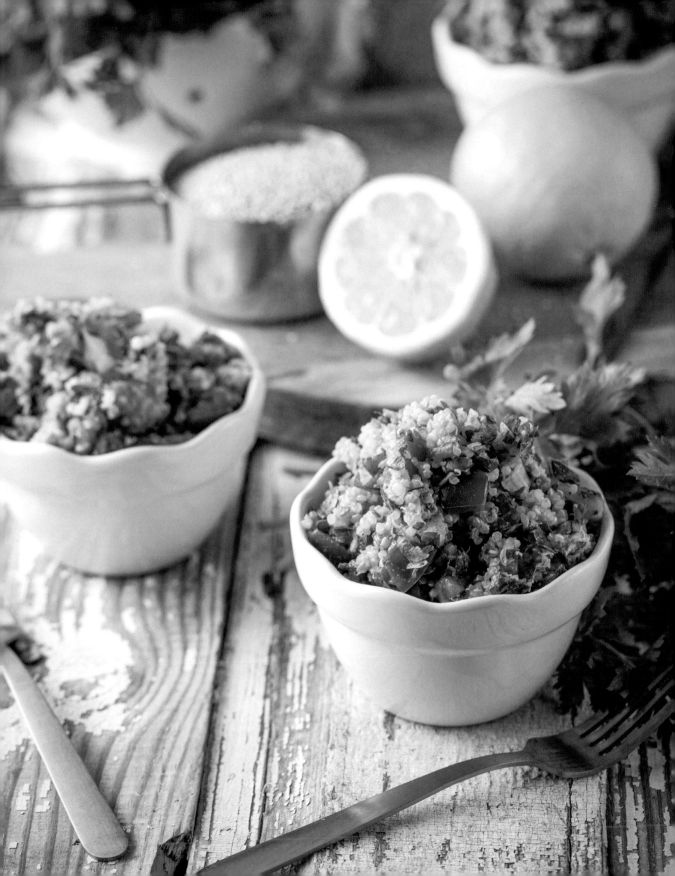

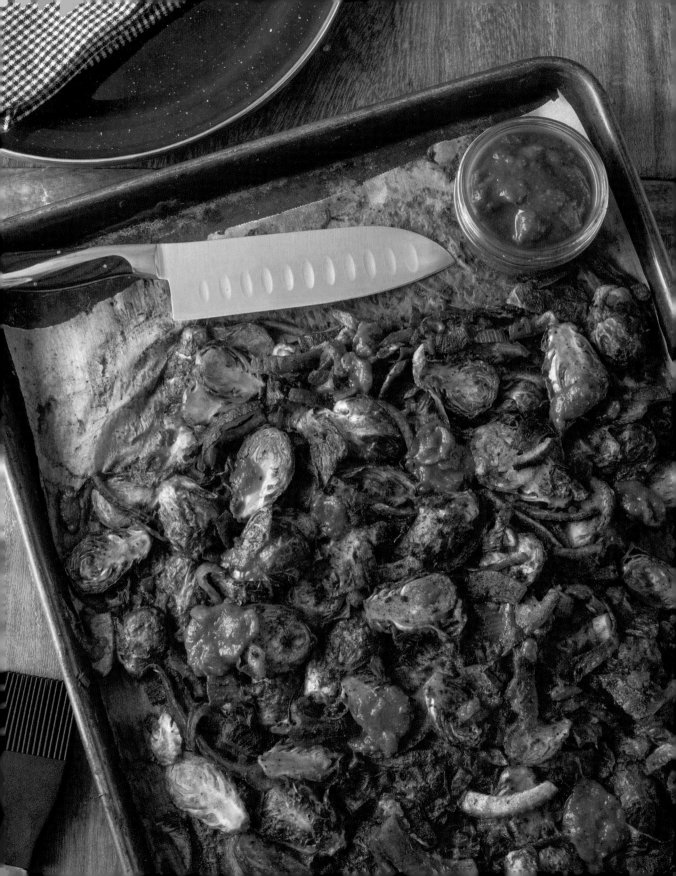

BBQ BRUSSELS SPROUTS

Who would have thought to combine barbecue and Brussels sprouts? We did! And the result is magnificent. This delectable dish is a hat tip to our hometown of Memphis, Tennessee, and our Peach BBQ Sauce really makes these veggies sing.

Yield: 4 cups | *Serves 4*

1 pound Brussels sprouts, sliced lengthwise into halves or quarters

1 medium red onion, sliced

1 tablespoon toasted sesame oil

½ teaspoon sea salt

½ teaspoon black pepper

1½ cups Peach BBQ Sauce (page 206)

1. Preheat your oven to 400°F.

2. Combine the Brussels sprouts, onion, sesame oil, salt, and pepper in a large mixing bowl.

3. Spread the Brussels sprouts mixture in a single layer on a parchment-lined baking sheet and bake for 20 minutes.

4. Drizzle the Brussels sprouts with the Peach BBQ Sauce, mix until evenly coated, and bake for another 10 minutes.

PRO TIP: Make it a meal by serving this atop Sweet Potato Grits (page 57).

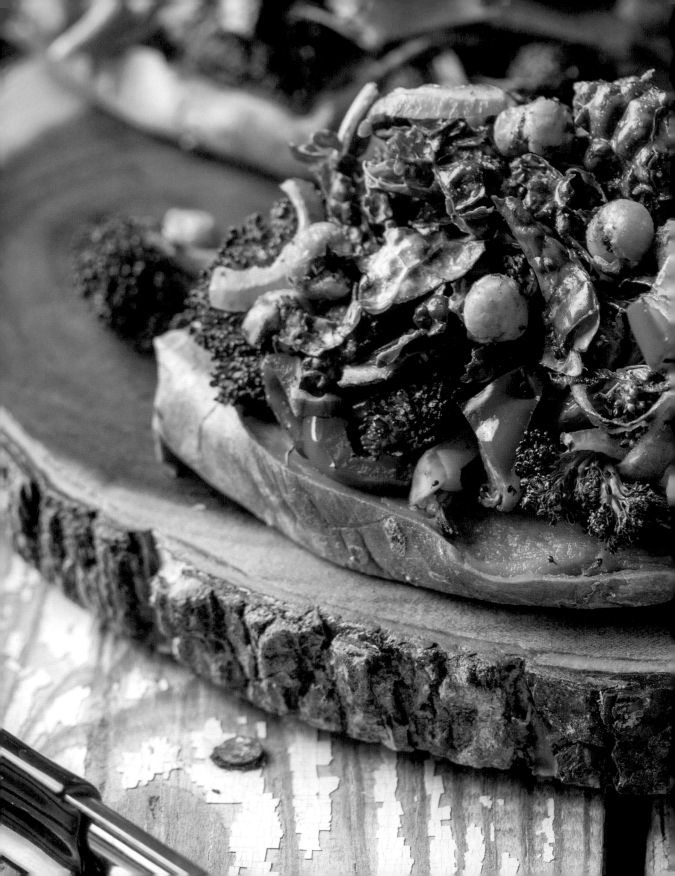

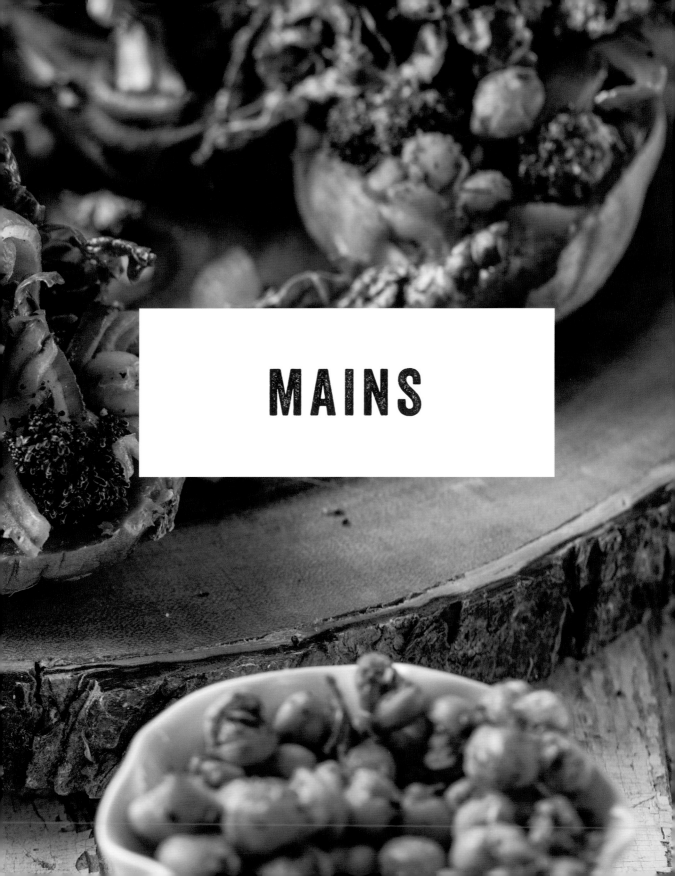

MAINS

CUBAN BLACK BEANS
with Baked Plantains

This dish is our salute to classic Cuban cuisine. Sweet roasted plantains accompany a rich savory stew of black beans with onions, peppers, and garlic. This is a super-hearty and satisfying dish with all the comfort-food feels.

Yield: 8 cups | *Serves 4 to 6*

Oven-Baked Plantains (recipe follows)

1 medium red onion, diced

1 tablespoon extra-virgin olive oil

1 medium red bell pepper, diced

1 medium green bell pepper, diced

1 medium head of garlic, peeled and sliced

1 medium jalapeño, seeded and minced

Two 15-ounce cans black beans with liquid, or 3 cups cooked beans with 1½ cups water or veggie broth

2 teaspoons maple syrup

1 tablespoon dried oregano

2 teaspoons cumin

1 teaspoon black pepper

2 bay leaves

1 tablespoon apple cider vinegar

½ teaspoon sea salt

2 medium avocados, sliced

Cilantro, to garnish

1. Make the Oven-Baked Plantains, baking them as you prepare the black beans.

2. Place the red onion and olive oil in a large stockpot over medium-high heat and cook for 5 minutes, or until the onion begins to soften.

3. Add the red and green bell peppers, garlic, jalapeño, black beans with their liquid, maple syrup, oregano, cumin, black pepper, bay leaves, vinegar, and salt.

4. Reduce the heat to medium-low, cover, and simmer for 20 minutes.

5. Serve in bowls topped with Baked Plantains, avocado, and cilantro.

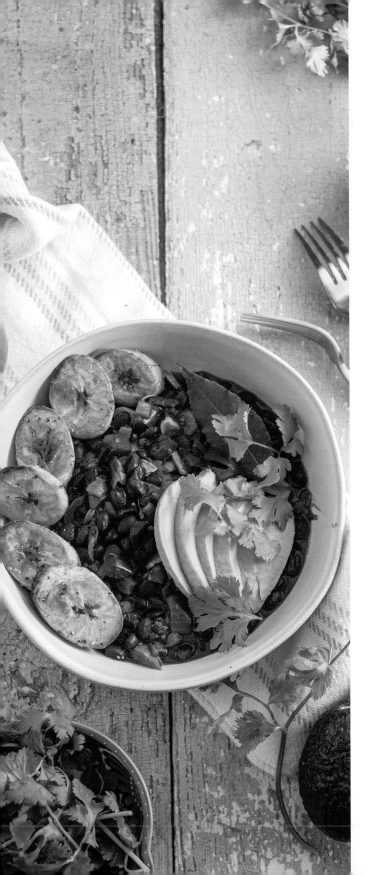

BAKED PLANTAINS

3 large ripe plantains
1½ tablespoons coconut oil or extra-virgin olive oil
Sea salt and black pepper, to taste

1. Preheat your oven to 350°F.

2. Peel and slice the plantains on the bias into ¼-inch slices.

3. Arrange the slices in a single layer on a parchment-lined baking sheet. Brush the plantains with oil and season with salt and pepper to taste.

4. Bake for 15 minutes.

5. Flip the plantains over and bake for another 15 to 20 minutes.

6. Serve warm as a snack or with the Cuban Black Beans.

NOTE: Do not use green plantains. The peel should be yellow and black, like an overripe banana. This will give you the perfect amount of starch and sweetness for this dish.

VEGGIE STIR-UP
with Orange-Ginger Sauce

This is a delicious assortment of our favorite anticancer veggies baked on a sheet pan with a classic Asian orange-ginger sauce. The end result is served over rice, similar to a stir-fry, but with much less oil. This dish is easy to whip up for a weeknight dinner.

Yield: 10 cups | *Serves 4*

2 cups black, red, or brown rice

1 medium bunch broccoli, broken into florets (about 6 cups)

1 medium red pepper, seeded and sliced

1 bunch green onions, white parts chopped into 1-inch pieces, tops sliced and reserved for garnish

One 8-ounce package shiitake mushrooms, sliced, woody part of the stem discarded

2 medium celery ribs, sliced

1 tablespoon toasted sesame oil

1 teaspoon Chinese five-spice powder

1 teaspoon black pepper

Orange-Ginger Sauce, divided (recipe follows)

1 cup cashews

1. Cook the rice according to the package instructions.

2. Preheat your oven to 375°F.

3. Mix and spread the broccoli, red pepper, white parts of the green onion, mushrooms, and celery on a large parchment-lined baking sheet.

4. Drizzle the sesame oil over the vegetables and add the Chinese five-spice and black pepper. Using your hands, toss the ingredients together and flatten them into a single layer.

5. Bake for 10 minutes, then remove from the oven and pour half of the Orange-Ginger Sauce onto the vegetables, tossing them using a spatula and flattening them back out into a single layer.

6. Bake for another 10 minutes.

7. Serve the veggies over rice. Garnish with cashews and the sliced green onion tops. Drizzle with the remaining Orange-Ginger Sauce to taste.

PRO TIP: Sheet-pan stir-ups are a great way to make use of random veggies in your fridge before they go to waste.

For more protein, add our Easy Baked Tofu (page 218).

For a completely different and delicious experience, try our Spicy Nut Butter Sauce (page 203) on these veggies instead of the Orange-Ginger Sauce.

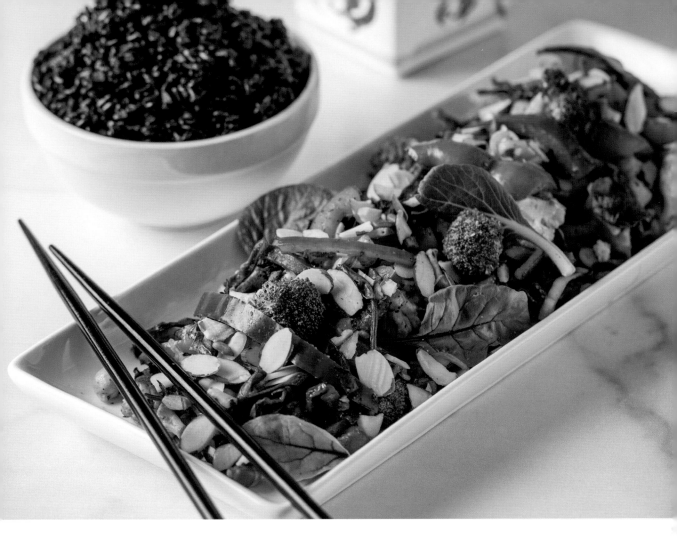

ORANGE-GINGER SAUCE

2 tablespoons unseasoned rice vinegar

Zest and juice of 2 medium oranges

2 tablespoons sriracha (optional)

4 tablespoons coconut aminos

2 teaspoons grated fresh ginger

1. Whisk together all the ingredients in a medium bowl.

2. Set aside in the fridge until ready to use.

PRO TIP: This sauce is a terrific marinade for the Easy Baked Tofu (page 218). Just drop the tofu into the marinade when it's hot out of your oven and it'll soak up all the flavor.

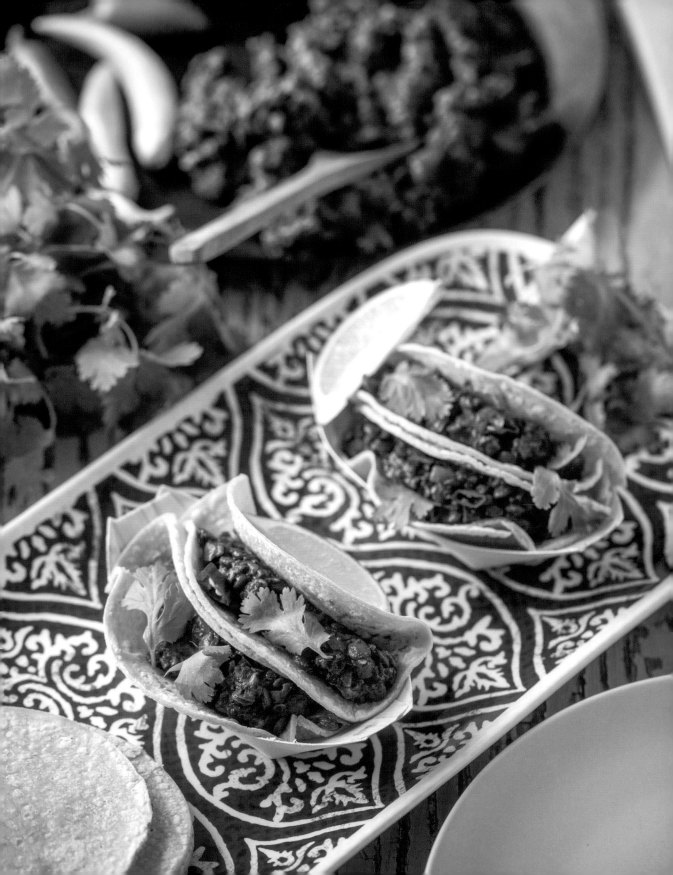

LENTIL TACOS

Lentils and walnuts are a nutritious and delicious ground beef substitute for tacos. The warmth of cumin, peppers, onion, and chili powder really makes the flavor pop. The whole family will love it. Perfect for Taco Tuesday!

Yield: 12 tacos | *Serves 4*

1 tablespoon toasted sesame oil or extra-virgin olive oil

1 medium red onion, diced

1 medium green bell pepper, diced

1 tablespoon chili powder

1 teaspoon cumin

½ teaspoon salt

½ cup dry lentils

½ cup finely chopped walnuts

3 cups low-sodium vegetable broth or Juicer Broth (page 214)

¼ cup (2 ounces) tomato paste

1 dozen small corn tortillas

1 cup loosely packed cilantro leaves

1 lime cut into wedges

Any other condiments you like on your taco like Juicer Hot Sauce (page 217) or Guac of Ages (page 192)

1. Place the oil, red onion, and bell pepper in a 12-inch cast-iron pan or heavy skillet over high heat and sauté for 5 to 7 minutes, or until most of the liquid has evaporated and the onion starts to brown.

2. Add the chili powder, cumin, salt, lentils, walnuts, and broth and reduce the heat to medium-low. Simmer uncovered for 20 minutes.

3. Add the tomato paste and continue to cook for another 5 minutes, or until the lentils are tender and the liquid has evaporated.

4. Serve warm stuffed into warmed tortillas topped with cilantro, a squeeze of lime, and any condiments of your choice.

NOTE: To make quick work of the chopping for this recipe, feel free to use your food processor.

PRO TIP: This lentil-and-walnut taco meat is perfect for tacos, but it's also fantastic on taco salads, rolled into enchiladas, tucked inside quesadillas, or even as a stand-alone side dish. Diced cherry tomatoes and sliced avocados also make great toppings.

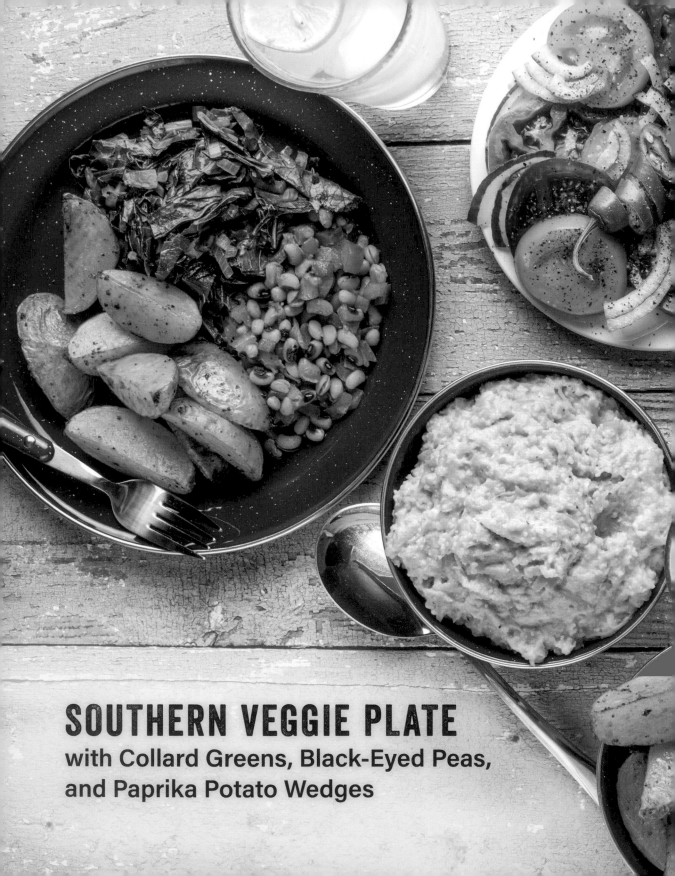

SOUTHERN VEGGIE PLATE
with Collard Greens, Black-Eyed Peas,
and Paprika Potato Wedges

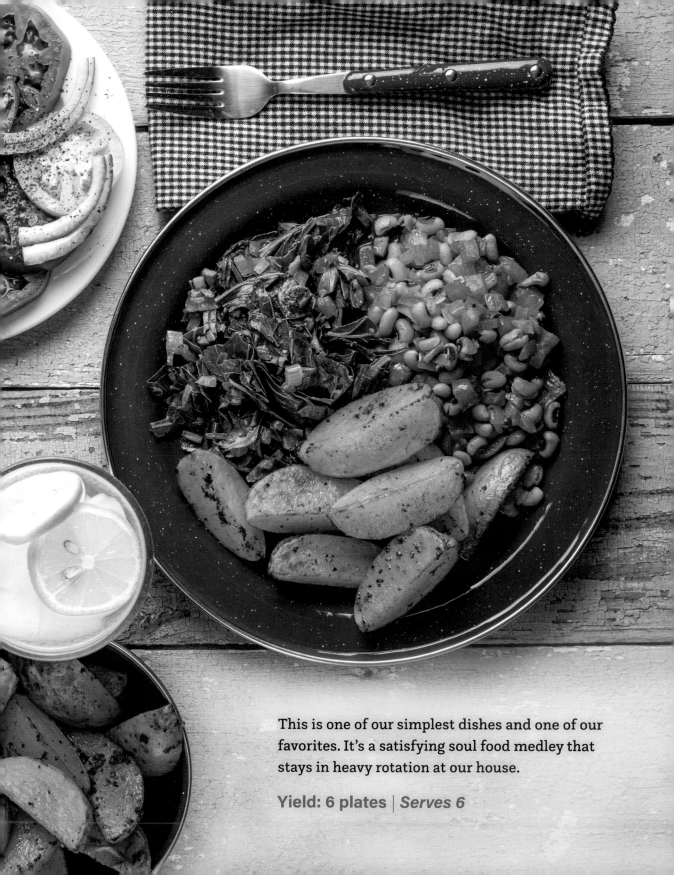

This is one of our simplest dishes and one of our favorites. It's a satisfying soul food medley that stays in heavy rotation at our house.

Yield: 6 plates | *Serves 6*

COLLARD GREENS

Yield: 3 to 4 cups | *Serves 6*

1 tablespoon extra-virgin olive oil

4 medium cremini mushrooms, diced

½ large white onion, diced

8 to 10 cups chopped collard green leaves, tough stems removed

½ teaspoon sea salt

½ teaspoon black pepper

2 teaspoons maple syrup

1½ cups water

1. Place the oil, mushrooms, and onion in a 12-inch cast-iron skillet over medium-high heat and sauté until the onion begins to brown.

2. Add the collard greens a handful at a time, wilting the greens before the next handful is added. Repeat until all the collard greens are added.

3. Reduce the heat to low and stir in the salt, pepper, maple syrup, and water. Cover and cook for 40 minutes, or until tender.

PRO TIP: To remove the tough stems from collard greens, fold the leaf in half lengthwise, holding both edges of the leaf in 1 hand, and use your other hand to pull the stem from the middle. It should break away from the leaf, leaving you holding the 2 halves of the leaf. Discard the stem.

BLACK-EYED PEAS

Yield: 3 cups | *Serves 6*

1 tablespoon extra-virgin olive oil

½ large white onion, diced

1 medium green bell pepper, diced

One 15-ounce can black-eyed peas with liquid, or 1½ cups cooked peas with 6 ounces water

1 tablespoon apple cider vinegar

½ teaspoon sea salt

½ teaspoon black pepper

2 tablespoons tomato paste

1. Place the olive oil, onion, and bell pepper in a medium saucepan over high heat and sauté for 5 minutes, or until the onion is translucent and beginning to brown.

2. Stir in the black-eyed peas, vinegar, salt, pepper, and tomato paste.

3. Bring to a boil and then lower the heat to a simmer. Cover and keep warm until ready to serve.

PAPRIKA POTATO WEDGES

Yield: 8 cups | *Serves 6*

2 pounds Yukon Gold potatoes, cut into wedges

1 tablespoon extra-virgin olive oil

1 tablespoon apple cider vinegar

½ teaspoon sea salt

½ teaspoon black pepper

1 teaspoon sweet paprika

1. Preheat your oven to 400°F.

2. Combine all the ingredients in a large mixing bowl and toss until the potatoes are evenly coated.

3. Spread the potatoes into a single layer on a parchment-lined baking sheet and bake for 20 minutes.

A meta-analysis of more than 180 observational studies and 50 clinical trials from the past 40 years found a 15 percent to 30 percent reduced risk of death and chronic disease in people who ate the most fiber, compared to those who ate the least. A fiber-rich diet was linked to a 22 percent lower risk of stroke, a 16 percent lower risk of type 2 diabetes, a 16 percent lower risk of colorectal cancer, and a 30 percent lower risk of death from heart disease.[61] To drop your risk, you need at least 30 grams of fiber per day. But fiber supplements aren't the solution. The majority of fiber studies are on people who consume fiber from whole-food sources: fruits, vegetables, legumes, nuts, seeds, and whole grains. You can easily consume more than 30 grams of fiber per day by eating a whole-food plant-based diet. The Southern Veggie Plate gives you 15 to 20 grams of fiber in one meal.

SWEET POTATO QUESADILLAS

Our quesadillas are stuffed with mashed sweet potato, black beans, roasted mushrooms, red peppers, and onions, spiced with cumin and coriander, and garnished with arugula and avocado. If your mouth is watering now, just wait until a quesadilla is on your plate!

Yield: 4 to 6 quesadillas | *Serves 4 to 6*

---

4 sweet potatoes

1 medium red bell pepper or 1 large poblano pepper, seeded and sliced

1 medium red onion, sliced

One-half 8-ounce package cremini mushrooms, sliced

1 teaspoon cumin

$\frac{1}{2}$ teaspoon ground coriander

1 teaspoon dried oregano

1 tablespoon extra-virgin olive oil

One 15-ounce can black beans, drained, or 1$\frac{1}{2}$ cups cooked beans

$\frac{1}{4}$ teaspoon sea salt

1 to 2 medium jalapeños, seeded and minced

$\frac{1}{2}$ cup nutritional yeast

Juice of 2 limes

4 to 6 large whole-grain tortillas

1 teaspoon extra-virgin olive oil

3 cups loosely packed arugula

2 medium avocados, sliced

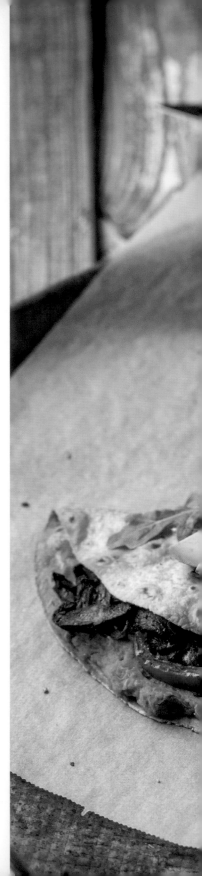

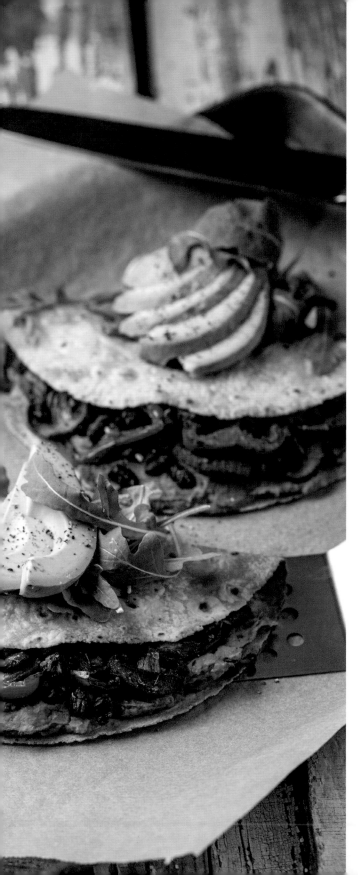

1. Preheat your oven to 400°F.

2. Place the sweet potatoes on a small baking sheet and bake for 40 minutes. Set aside.

3. Mix the bell pepper, onion, mushrooms, cumin, coriander, oregano, and olive oil on a large, parchment-lined baking sheet and bake for 20 minutes. This can be done in the same oven in tandem with the baking of the sweet potatoes. Remove the vegetables from your oven, toss in the black beans and ¼ teaspoon sea salt and set aside. (Keep your oven at 400°F for baking the quesadillas.)

4. Mash the skin-on sweet potatoes with the jalapeño, nutritional yeast, and lime juice in a medium bowl.

5. Spread ½ cup of the sweet potato mixture evenly over half of each tortilla, top the sweet potato mixture with ½ cup vegetable and beans mixture, and fold each into a half-circle.

6. Place the quesadillas in a single layer on 1 or 2 parchment-lined baking sheets and brush the tops lightly with oil. Bake the quesadillas for 10 minutes, flip over, and bake another 5 minutes, or until golden brown.

7. Garnish each quesadilla with ½ cup arugula and sliced avocado.

JERK PINEAPPLE STEAKS

This is our homage to much-loved Jamaican jerk dishes with pineapple taking center stage. Prepare your taste buds for a sweet and savory tropical delight spiced with chili peppers, garlic, nutmeg, allspice, and ginger over a bed of red beans and rice. Yum!

Yield: 10 cups | *Serves 4 to 6*

---

2 medium serrano chili peppers, seeds and ribs removed

8 medium green onions, root ends trimmed

1-inch piece of fresh ginger

3 cups loose-packed parsley, plus more for garnish

2 tablespoons fresh thyme leaves, plus more for garnish

Zest and juice of 2 medium limes

8 medium garlic cloves

2 teaspoons allspice

1 teaspoon black pepper

¼ teaspoon nutmeg

2 tablespoons coconut aminos

2 tablespoons extra-virgin olive oil

One 13.5-ounce can light coconut milk

Two 15.5-ounce cans red beans or pigeon peas with liquid, or 3 cups cooked beans

1 cup long-grain brown rice

½ teaspoon sea salt

1 medium pineapple, peeled and sliced into 6 slices

1. Preheat your oven to 375°F.

2. Blend the serrano peppers, green onions, ginger, parsley, thyme, lime zest and juice, garlic, allspice, pepper, nutmeg, coconut aminos, and olive oil in the work bowl of a food processor until well mixed. This makes about 1 cup of jerk paste.

3. Place the coconut milk, beans with their liquid, rice, salt, and half of the jerk paste in a 12-inch round pan or a 9 x 12-inch casserole dish and mix together.

4. Shingle the pineapple slices on top of the mixture and brush the pineapple with the remaining jerk paste.

5. Bake for 30 minutes, then gently stir the rice mixture around the pineapple slices and bake for another 10 minutes.

6. Serve hot, garnished with parsley and thyme.

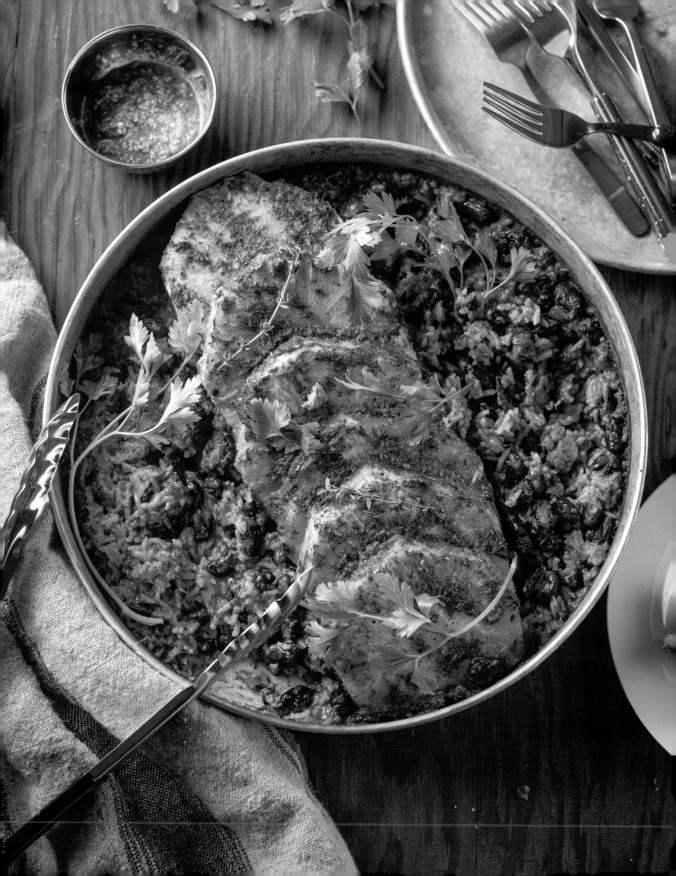

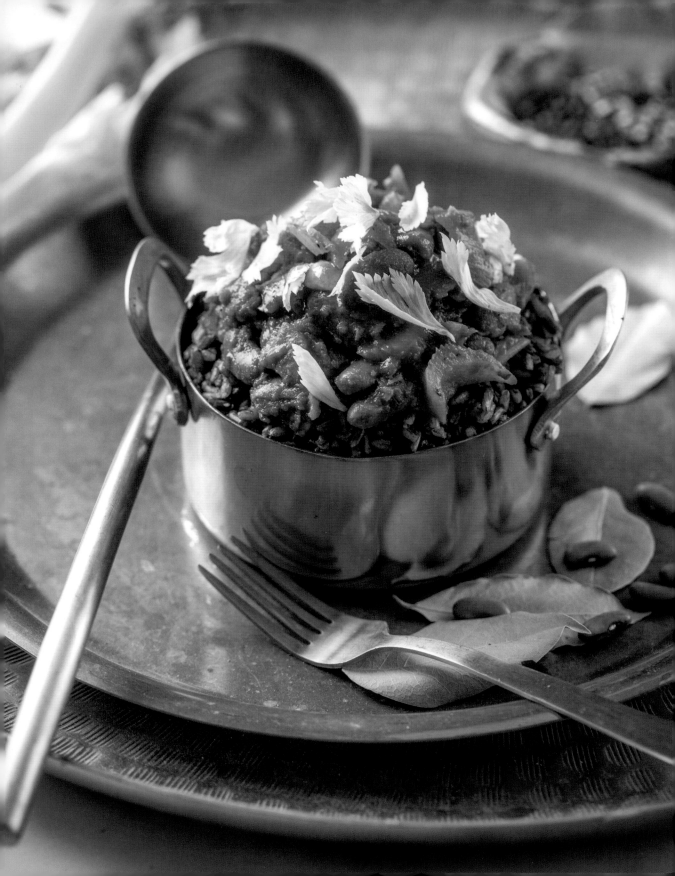

RED BEANS AND RED RICE

Get into that funky New Orleans vibe with our porkless beans and rice, jazzed up with anti-cancer spices. This dish always hits the spot.

Yield: 10 cups | *Serves 6 to 8*

4 cups red rice

1 tablespoon extra-virgin olive oil

2 cups diced yellow onion (from about 1 large)

1½ cups sliced celery (from about 3 ribs)

1 medium green bell pepper, diced

8 garlic cloves, minced

½ teaspoon crushed red pepper

½ teaspoon paprika

1 teaspoon dried thyme

1 teaspoon black pepper

½ teaspoon sea salt

2 bay leaves

One 28-ounce can crushed tomatoes

Two 15-ounce cans dark red kidney beans with liquid

1 tablespoon mustard

1 tablespoon apple cider vinegar

Chopped celery leaves, to garnish

1. Cook the rice according to the package instructions.

2. Sauté the olive oil, onion, and celery in a stockpot over high heat for 5 minutes, or until the onion turns translucent.

3. Reduce the heat to medium. Add the bell pepper, garlic, crushed red pepper, paprika, thyme, black pepper, and salt to the pot and cook for 3 minutes, stirring often.

4. Stir in the bay leaves, tomatoes, beans, mustard, and vinegar. Reduce the heat to a simmer and cook uncovered for 20 minutes.

5. Serve the beans over the rice, garnished with chopped celery leaves and a few dashes of hot sauce, if desired.

PRO TIP: Celery leaves make a terrific garnish and are full of flavor. Use the tender, small celery leaves at the center of each celery stalk.

CABBAGE ROAST

This is a great dish for holidays and family get-togethers and is an excellent way to get more cruciferous cabbage into your life. The root vegetables and mushrooms create a natural au jus that is bursting with flavor. Perfect as a side or main course.

Yield: 4 slices | *Serves 4*

1 pound baby gold potatoes

1 medium onion, chopped

One 8-ounce package cremini mushrooms, quartered

4 medium carrots, peeled and cut into 1-inch pieces

1 medium cabbage, sliced into 4 pieces with the stem end intact

2 tablespoons toasted sesame oil

2 tablespoons apple cider vinegar

¼ cup orange juice

1 tablespoon maple syrup

½ teaspoon black pepper

3 tablespoons coconut aminos

Fresh herbs, such as a few sprigs of parsley, sage, thyme, or rosemary, plus more for garnish

Salt, to taste

1. Preheat your oven to 400°F.

2. Mix the potatoes, onion, mushrooms, and carrots in a Dutch oven or a 9 x 13-inch casserole dish with a cover.

3. Shingle the cabbage steaks atop the mixed vegetables.

4. Whisk the sesame oil, vinegar, orange juice, maple syrup, black pepper, and coconut aminos in a medium bowl, then drizzle the mixture atop the cabbage and vegetables.

5. Top with fresh herbs, tightly cover the dish, and bake for 1½ hours.

6. Remove and discard the herbs, and bake uncovered for an additional 15 minutes.

7. Transfer the vegetables to a serving platter, but do not throw out the juice that has accumulated at the bottom of the dish. Garnish with fresh herbs and pour the juice over the top of the cabbage. Salt to taste.

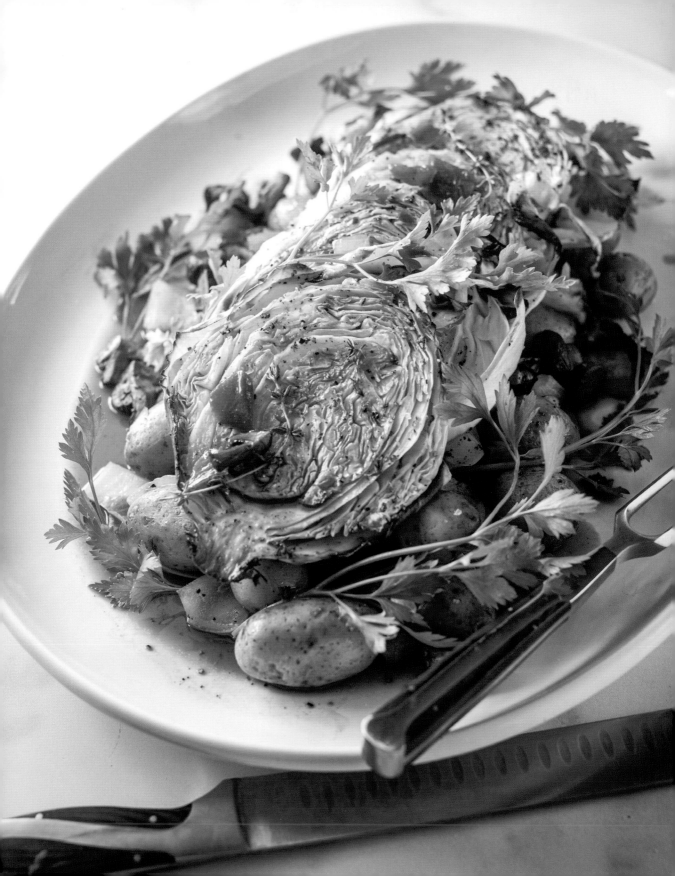

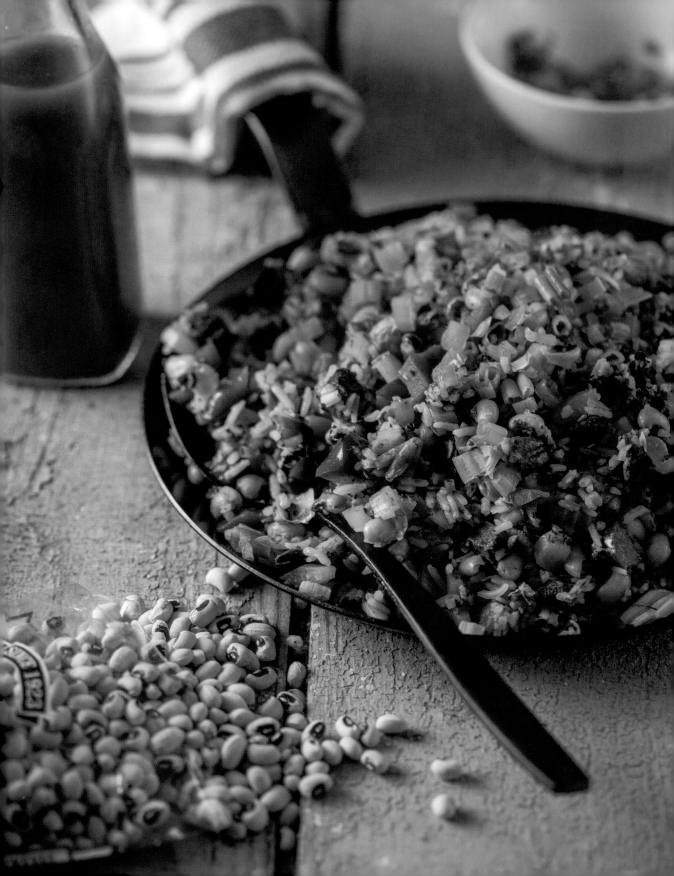

HOPPIN' JOHN

Our Hoppin' John is a black-eyed peas and rice dish with mushrooms, peppers, celery, onions, and savory spices. It's a southern tradition to eat black-eyed peas on New Year's Day for good luck. This dish might just bring you a little extra. Be ready with all the ingredients because this cooks fast!

Yield: 5 cups | *Serves 4*

1 tablespoon toasted sesame oil

1 large portobello mushroom, diced

2 cups cooked and cooled long-grain brown rice

1½ cups cooked black-eyed peas, drained and rinsed

1 medium red bell pepper, diced

2 medium celery ribs, diced

1 bunch green onions, sliced, tops and white parts separated

½ teaspoon sea salt

¼ teaspoon black pepper

¼ teaspoon granulated garlic

½ teaspoon dried thyme

1 to 2 tablespoons apple cider vinegar

1. Preheat a large wok or large frying pan over high heat.

2. Add the sesame oil to the hot pan, and once the oil shimmers, add the mushroom and cook for 30 seconds.

3. Add the rice, peas, bell pepper, celery, white part of the green onions, salt, pepper, garlic, thyme, and vinegar, all while constantly moving the mixture around the pan.

4. Continue to stir and cook for about 4 to 5 minutes, or until everything is heated through but the vegetables retain some crunch.

5. Serve warm, garnished with green onion tops.

PRO TIP: Sprinkle with our Juicer Hot Sauce (page 217) to give it a little kick.

OVERSTUFFED SWEET POTATOES

Here's the plan: Load up a sweet potato with roasted anticancer veggies and savory spices and devour. A happy belly awaits . . .

Yield: 6 stuffed potato halves | *Serves 3 to 6*

---

3 medium sweet potatoes

1 medium red onion, sliced

1 medium bunch broccolini, sliced

1 medium red bell pepper, sliced

1 tablespoon sesame oil

¼ teaspoon sea salt

¼ teaspoon black pepper

Juice of 1 medium lemon

1 bunch kale, stems removed

2 tablespoons tahini

1 tablespoon maple syrup

1 cup Shake & Bake Chickpeas (page 220)

1. Preheat your oven to 400°F.

2. Massage the lemon juice into the kale in a medium bowl, tearing and ripping the kale leaves into bite-size pieces. Allow this to rest for 10 minutes.

3. Bake the sweet potatoes on a small baking sheet for 40 minutes. Set aside. Allow to rest for at least 20 minutes.

4. Spread the onion, broccolini, and bell pepper on a large, parchment-lined baking sheet. Drizzle with sesame oil, season with salt and pepper, and bake for 20 minutes. This can be done in the same oven in tandem with the baking of the sweet potatoes.

5. Add the tahini and maple syrup to the kale and toss to coat.

6. Cut the warm sweet potatoes in half, topping them with the roasted vegetables and kale, and lastly with the chickpeas.

PRO TIP: Before cooking, allow cruciferous veggies like broccoli and kale to sit for 20 to 40 minutes after slicing, chopping, or tearing. During this time, a special enzymatic reaction takes place, which creates the anticancer compound sulforaphane.

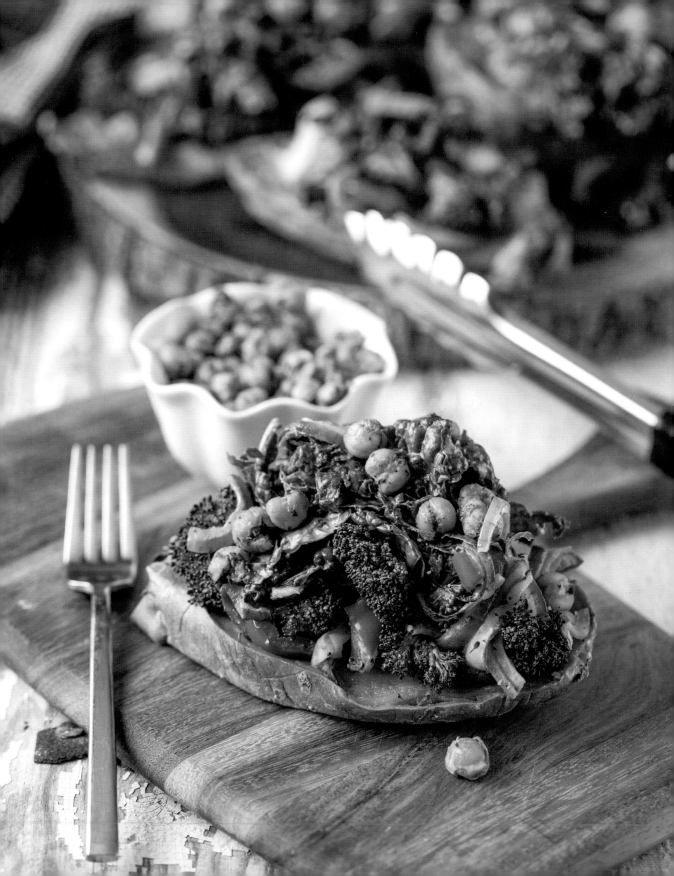

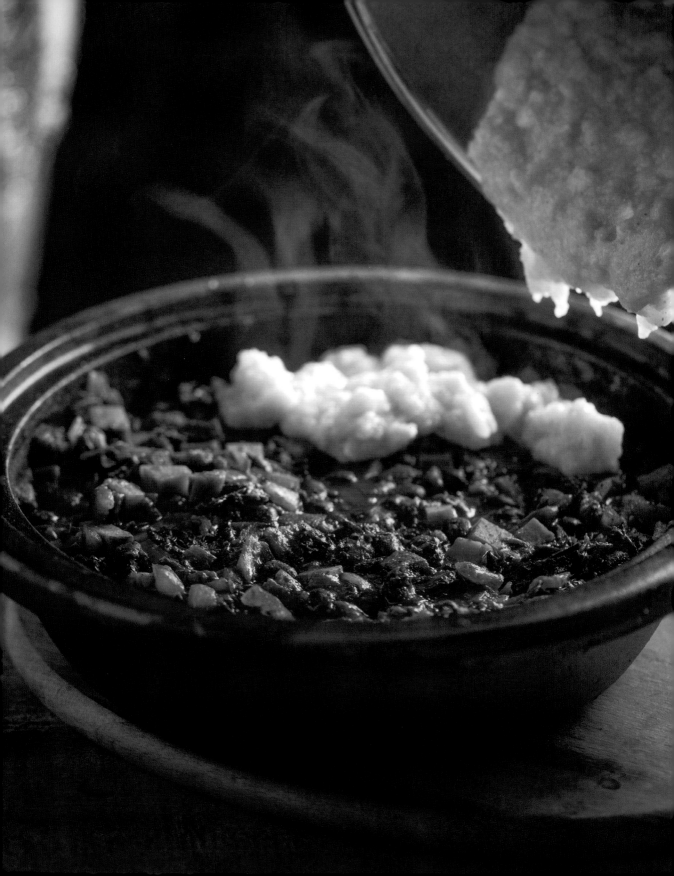

TAMALE PIE

Our tamale pie delivers the dynamic duo of sweet potatoes and black beans in a spicy tomato sauce topped with a warm corn crust. This super-easy dish delivers all the tamale flavor without all the work of making tamales.

Yield: 8 cups | *Serves 4 to 6*

1 tablespoon extra-virgin olive oil

1 medium red onion, diced

1 bunch kale, de-stemmed and chopped

1 small sweet potato, diced

2 teaspoons cumin

1 teaspoon ground coriander

½ teaspoon granulated garlic

½ teaspoon sea salt

One 15-ounce can black beans with liquid

One 14.5-ounce can diced tomatoes with liquid

2 cups low-sodium vegetable broth, such as Juicer Broth (page 214)

½ cup cornmeal

1 cup corn kernels (from about 1 large ear of corn)

1 large jalapeño pepper, thinly sliced

Guacamole, to garnish

1. Preheat your oven to 350°F.

2. Sauté the olive oil and onion in a large cast-iron skillet or frying pan over high heat for 3 minutes, or until the onion has softened.

3. Add the kale and stir until the kale has wilted.

4. Stir in the sweet potato, cumin, coriander, garlic, salt, black beans, and tomatoes until heated through, and then turn off the heat.

5. Whisk the broth, cornmeal, and corn kernels in a medium saucepan over high heat until the mixture comes to a boil and thickens.

6. Pour the corn mixture evenly atop the vegetables, layer with jalapeño slices, and bake for 30 minutes.

7. Let the pie cool for 10 minutes. Serve warm with guacamole to garnish.

Black beans are among the highest-antioxidant beans and have shown potent antiproliferative activity against breast, colon, and liver cancer cells.[62]

STUFFED SPAGHETTI SQUASH

Warm spaghetti squash right out of your oven, stuffed with chunky tomato sauce, carrots, onions, peppers, white beans, and celery, and garnished with whole roasted garlic cloves. It can all be yours tonight.

Serves 6

3 small spaghetti squash, halved lengthwise and seeds scraped out

2 medium heads of garlic, top ⅓ cut off

2 tablespoons extra-virgin olive oil, divided

½ teaspoon sea salt

2 medium celery ribs, sliced

3 medium carrots, sliced

1 medium white onion, diced

1 medium green bell pepper, diced

One 8-ounce package cremini mushrooms, sliced

One 28-ounce can diced tomatoes

One 14.5-ounce can crushed tomatoes

One 15-ounce can cannellini beans with liquid

½ teaspoon crushed red pepper

1 tablespoon Italian seasoning or Bragg Organic Sprinkle

1 tablespoon champagne vinegar or red wine vinegar

Chopped parsley and No Harm Parm (page 196), to garnish

1. Preheat your oven to 400°F.

2. Place the spaghetti squash and the garlic, cut side up, on a large, parchment-lined baking sheet, drizzle with 1 tablespoon olive oil, and sprinkle with salt.

3. Bake for 30 minutes, during which time you may make the sauce.

4. Place the remaining tablespoon of olive oil in a large skillet over high heat. Add the celery, carrots, and onion and sauté until the onion is translucent, about 5 minutes.

5. Stir in the bell pepper, mushrooms, diced and crushed tomatoes, beans, crushed red pepper, Italian seasoning, and vinegar until the mixture heats through.

6. Once the spaghetti squash and garlic are baked, hold the hot squash with tongs and carefully scrape the flesh away from the skin to form a mound, keeping the skin intact.

7. Divide the sauce among the cooked squash in the skins. Really pile it on!

8. Serve warm, garnished with parsley, No Harm Parm, and some roasted garlic cloves.

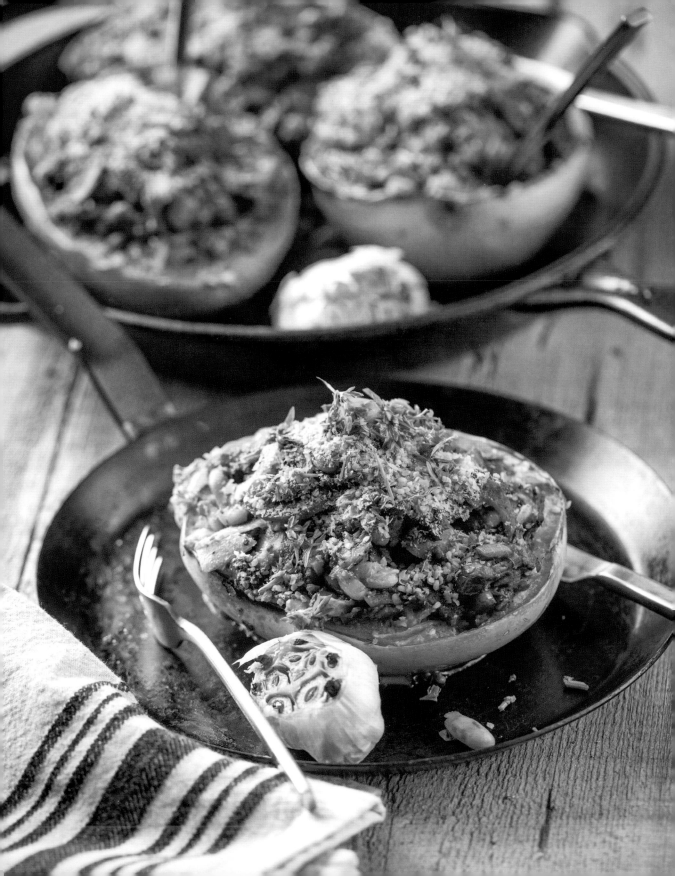

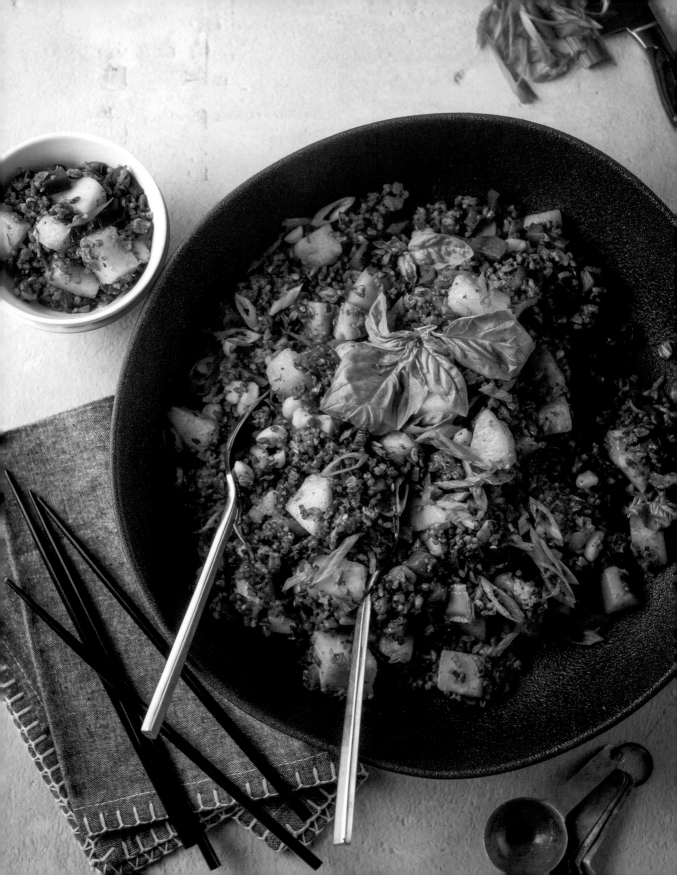

PINEAPPLE AND BASIL RICE

Our non-fried version of Thai fried rice, combining the sweetness of pineapple with spicy hot peppers and aromatic notes of basil, is simply delightful. This is one of our favorite dishes in the whole book! Have all ingredients ready to go because this cooks quickly.

Yield: 8 cups | *Serves 4*

1 tablespoon toasted sesame oil

3 medium garlic cloves, minced

1 teaspoon fresh ginger, grated

3 cups pineapple chunks

1 medium red bell pepper, diced

½ cup macadamia nuts

1 medium serrano pepper, minced (optional)

1 bunch green onions, sliced, darker green tops reserved for garnish

3 cups cooked and cooled red rice

Juice and zest of 1 lime

1 tablespoon coconut aminos, plus more to drizzle

1 bunch basil leaves, thinly sliced (about ½ cup)

NOTE: This is perfect with any leftover rice. If you don't have leftover rice, make sure to cook and cool the rice before you start this recipe. Warm rice will stick to the pan and turn out gummy.

1. Sauté the oil, garlic, and ginger in a wok or large frying pan over high heat for about 30 seconds.

2. Add the pineapple, bell pepper, macadamia nuts, serrano pepper, white and light green parts of the green onions, rice, lime juice and zest, and coconut aminos, constantly tossing the ingredients. Alternately, use a large spoon if you're not comfortable with the pan flip.

3. Cook 4 to 5 minutes, or until everything is heated through.

4. Drizzle coconut aminos over the top and garnish with basil.

NOTE: To bulk up this meal, add 1 to 2 cups of cooked black beans or chickpeas in Step 2.

Pineapples contain an anti-inflammatory, anticancer enzyme called bromelain, which has been shown to suppress the growth of many types of cancer cells and improve anticancer immune function.[63]

DIY SUSHI TACOS

This is a fun do-it-yourself option where everyone creates their own unique sushi experience. To make it super easy, we layer the ingredients on a small nori sheet and scoop it up taco-style.

Yield: 24 pieces | *Serves 4*

1 tablespoon toasted sesame oil

1 tablespoon coconut aminos

1 garlic clove, minced

2 tablespoons grated ginger

One 8-ounce package shiitake mushrooms, sliced

1 bunch asparagus, woody ends trimmed

1 medium carrot, shredded

1 small cucumber, cut into matchsticks

1 medium bunch basil, tough stems discarded

3 green onions, trimmed and sliced lengthwise

½ cup kimchi or sauerkraut

1 medium avocado, sliced

5 cups Maple Sushi Rice (page 219)

1 tablespoon (½ ounce) wasabi

Coconut aminos and sriracha, to taste

6 sheets of toasted nori, cut into quarters

1. Preheat your oven to 350°F.

2. To create the marinade, whisk the sesame oil, coconut aminos, garlic, and ginger in a medium mixing bowl.

3. Spread the mushrooms and asparagus on a parchment-lined baking sheet, brush them with the marinade, and bake for 20 minutes.

4. Transfer the mushroom-asparagus mixture to a large platter, and arrange the carrot, cucumber, basil, onions, kimchi, avocado, and Maple Sushi Rice in individual sections. Serve wasabi, coconut aminos, sriracha, and nori on the side.

5. Each diner can make their own combination by topping the nori with rice and a selection of vegetables and herbs. Pick it up taco-style for a casual sushi experience.

Nori is a seaweed rich in vitamins and minerals, including vitamins A, B_1, B_2, and C, plus potassium, magnesium, iron, zinc, and iodine.

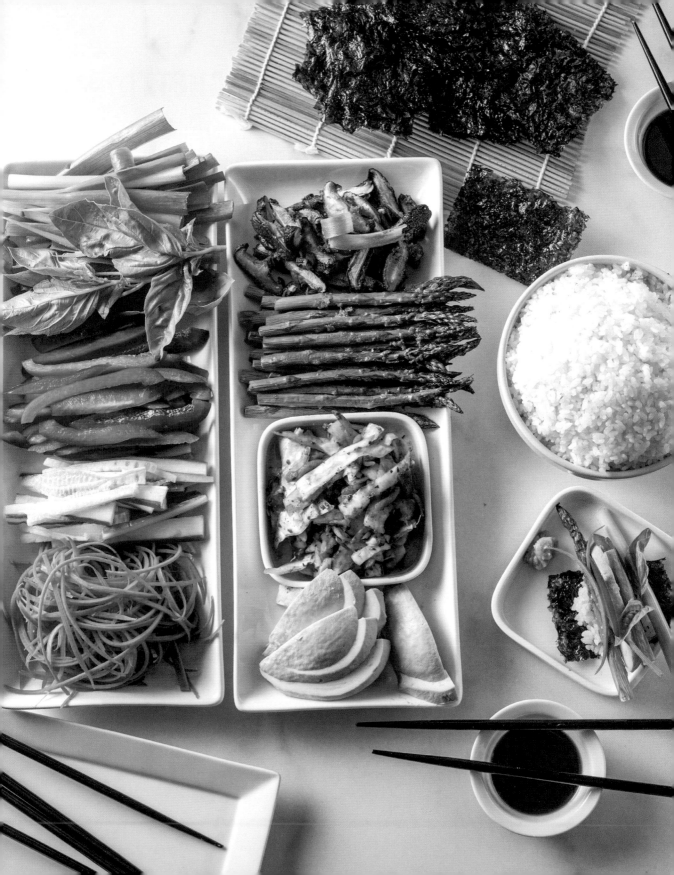

CAULIFLOWER AND KALE SPAGHETTI

Our cauliflower and almond sauce with rosemary is a rich and creamy plant-based alternative to Alfredo sauce and takes spaghetti to new heights. We adore this dish.

Yield: 6 cups | *Serves 4*

1 medium head of cauliflower, broken into florets and stem roughly chopped (about 5 cups)

10 medium garlic cloves

1 tablespoon extra-virgin olive oil

1 bunch curly kale, stems discarded and leafy parts roughly chopped

Juice and zest of 1 medium lemon

½ cup raw cashews

¼ teaspoon sea salt

½ teaspoon crushed red pepper

1 sprig fresh rosemary leaves, stem discarded

1 teaspoon maple syrup

1 pound dry whole-grain thin spaghetti or pasta of choice

½ cup toasted sliced almonds

1. Preheat your oven to 400°F.

2. Spread the cauliflower and garlic in a single layer on a parchment-lined baking sheet, drizzle with olive oil, and bake for 15 to 20 minutes, or until the edges start to brown.

3. Turn off the oven. Set aside the garlic and 1 cup of the cauliflower. Add the kale to the baking sheet and place it back in the oven. The residual heat will wilt the kale.

4. Using a food processor, blend the cauliflower and garlic previously set aside, along with the lemon juice and zest, cashews, salt, 1 cup of water, crushed red pepper, rosemary, and maple syrup until smooth. Wait 5 minutes and then blend for an additional 2 minutes. This will result in a smooth sauce without having to soak the cashews.

5. Cook the spaghetti in a large stockpot. Drain and return the spaghetti to the pot. Add the sauce to the pasta and cook over medium heat until it is warmed through.

6. Add the remaining cauliflower and kale to the pot and toss until the pasta is well coated with the sauce.

7. Garnish with sliced almonds and serve family style.

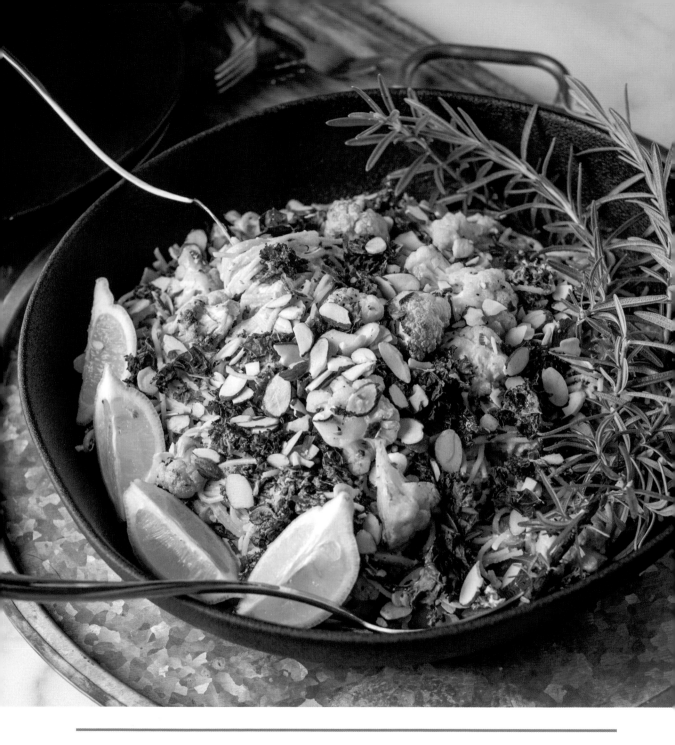

Raw and cooked kale have both been demonstrated to be immune boosters, significantly increasing IgM antibody production, your body's first line of defense against infections.[64]

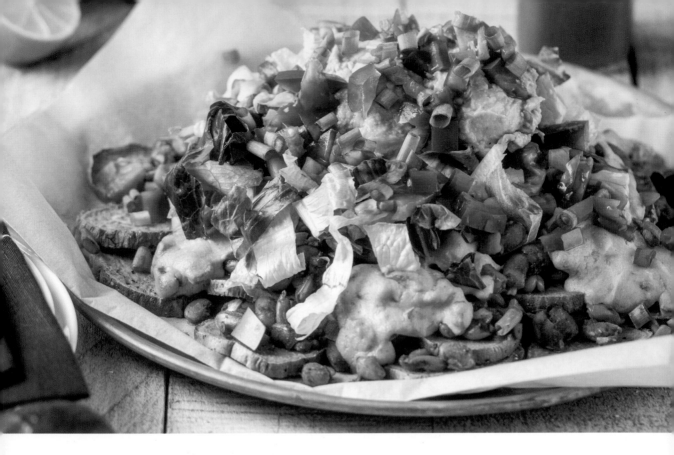

NACHO-STYLE SWEET POTATOES

This is how we do nachos. No cheese or tortilla chips needed!

Yield: One 10-inch tray | *Serves 2 as a main dish or 4 as a side or appetizer*

1 tablespoon extra-virgin olive oil

3 small sweet potatoes, sliced into ⅛-inch rounds

¼ teaspoon sea salt

¼ teaspoon black pepper

One 15-ounce can pinto beans, drained, or 1½ cups cooked beans

½ teaspoon cumin

½ teaspoon ground coriander

½ teaspoon dried oregano

1 tablespoon sweet paprika

½ medium onion, diced (about ½ cup)

1 large jalapeño pepper, seeds removed and finely diced

1 tablespoon apple cider vinegar

1 cup Nacho Cheeze Dip (page 209)

1 heaping cup shredded red romaine or other leafy green

¼ cup chopped chives or green onions

1 medium Roma tomato, diced

½ cup Super-Fresh Salsa (page 195)

1 cup Guac of Ages (page 192)

1. Toss the olive oil, sweet potatoes, salt, and pepper in a large mixing bowl.

2. Spread the potatoes in a single layer on 2 parchment-lined sheet pans. Keep the bowl out for Step 5.

3. Place the sheet pans into a cold oven. Set the oven to 400°F and bake for 20 minutes.

4. Remove the potatoes and allow to cool slightly, but keep your oven on.

5. Combine the beans, cumin, coriander, oregano, paprika, onion, jalapeño, and vinegar in the large mixing bowl used for the potatoes.

6. Top 1 of the sheet pans of sweet potatoes with $1/2$ of the bean mixture. Spread the remaining potatoes over the beans and top with the remaining bean mixture.

7. Top with the Nacho Cheeze Dip and bake for 10 minutes to warm through.

8. Garnish with red romaine, chives, tomatoes, salsa, and guacamole.

Oregano is an antimicrobial, anti-inflammatory, anticancer spice. It is one of the highest-antioxidant spices on earth, and one teaspoon of oregano has the same antioxidant power as two cups of red grapes. Oregano contains the flavonoid quercetin, which is known to slow cancer growth and promote apoptosis. It also contains vitamin K and iron. Laboratory studies have found oregano extracts to cause cancer cell death in colon cancer, breast cancer, and prostate cancer.[65,66,67]

THE BETA BURGER

Instead of store bought veggie burgers, which are heavily processed with high levels of sodium, we suggest making your own. Our savory Beta Burger patty is made from mushrooms and oats, two of the best sources of beta glucans, a special type of immune boosting fiber that is anticancer, antimicrobial, and even shown to reduce the risk of cardiovascular disease. Also known as the World's Best Mushroom Oat Burger.

Yield: 6 burgers | *Serves 6*

1 pound cremini or white button mushrooms

2 teaspoons sea salt

1 tablespoon apple cider vinegar

3 cups rolled oats

2 teaspoons black pepper

2 to 3 tablespoons extra-virgin olive oil, divided

6 sprouted whole-grain hamburger buns or 6 large lettuce leaves

Mustard, Lemony Almond Hummus (page 191), pickles, red onions, sliced tomato, lettuce, and avocado, for garnish

PRO TIP: Make sure your patties have smooth, rounded edges. This makes them less likely to fall apart as they cook.

This recipe can also be used to make meatballs for spaghetti.

Excess estrogen is harmful and can fuel cancer growth. Aromatase is an enzyme that converts testosterone into estrogen in the body. White button mushrooms have been found to suppress aromatase by 60 percent, better than any other vegetable or mushroom tested.[68] In addition, eating one cup of cooked white button mushrooms per day has been shown to accelerate the salivary secretion of an immune system antibody called immunoglobulin A by 50 percent.[69]

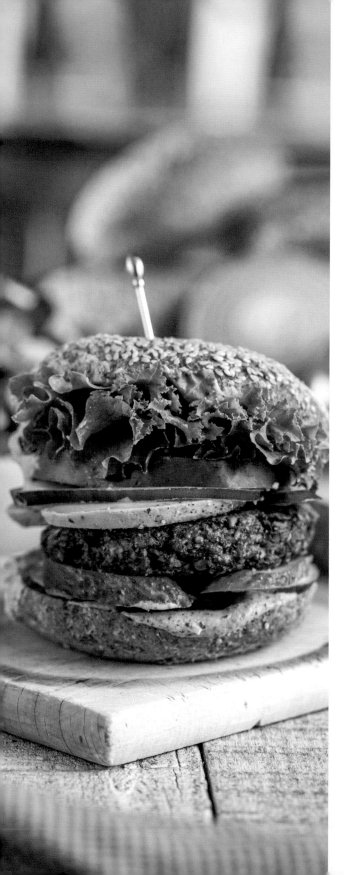

1. Pulse the mushrooms in the work bowl of your food processor until they are finely chopped but not blended. Work in batches as needed.

2. Combine the chopped mushrooms and salt in a large mixing bowl. Allow the mixture to rest for 5 minutes. You'll notice that the water is being pulled from the mushrooms; do not discard that water!

3. Add the vinegar, oats, and pepper. Using your hands, knead the mushrooms and oats together until well incorporated. The mix will seem a little dry at first.

4. Cover with plastic wrap and refrigerate for 20 minutes.

5. Knead the mixture once more. This time, it should resemble ground beef—seriously! Divide the mixture into 6 equal balls.

6. Press each ball into roughly a 4-inch patty on a sheet of parchment or wax paper.

7. Place 1½ tablespoons of olive oil in a large cast-iron skillet or frying pan set over medium heat. Pan-fry the burgers 3 at a time for about 4 minutes per side. Add the remaining oil before cooking the second batch.

8. Serve hot on a toasted bun or over lettuce, topped however you'd like.

BEAN BREAD PESTO PIZZA

This is how we do pizza. No cheese, loaded with veggies, and super delish. Our homemade pizza crust made from garbanzo beans and rice is a terrific option for a homemade gluten-free pizza crust.

Yield: One 12-inch pizza | *Serves 2 to 4*

Bean Bread Batter

½ cup rice flour

1 cup garbanzo bean flour

½ teaspoon sea salt

2 ¼ teaspoons (1 packet) rapid-rise yeast

1 ¼ cups water

2 teaspoons extra-virgin olive oil

Pizza Toppings

½ cup sliced broccoli

½ cup sliced bell pepper

½ cup sliced cauliflower

½ cup sliced zucchini

¼ cup diced onion

1 tablespoon extra-virgin olive oil

1 tablespoon balsamic vinegar

1 teaspoon Italian seasoning

½ cup Broccoli Sprout Pesto (page 188)*

½ cup No Harm Parm (page 196)

Crushed red pepper flakes, to taste

1. Preheat your oven to 425°F.

2. Whisk all the ingredients for the Bean Bread Batter in a large mixing bowl until there are no lumps, about the same consistency as pancake batter.

3. Coat a large, 15-inch parchment-lined pizza pan with olive oil.

4. Add the Bean Bread Batter, shake the pan to form an even circle, set aside, and allow the batter to rise for 20 minutes.

5. Bake the crust for 10 minutes, or until it just starts to turn golden brown.

6. Toss the broccoli, bell pepper, cauliflower, zucchini, onion, olive oil, vinegar, and Italian seasoning in a large mixing bowl until the vegetables are evenly coated.

7. Spread the pesto onto the crust in a thin layer. Add the vegetable mixture in an even layer. Bake for an additional 20 minutes.

8. Slice the pizza and sprinkle with No Harm Parm and crushed red pepper flakes.

*Feel free to substitute tomato sauce for the pesto.

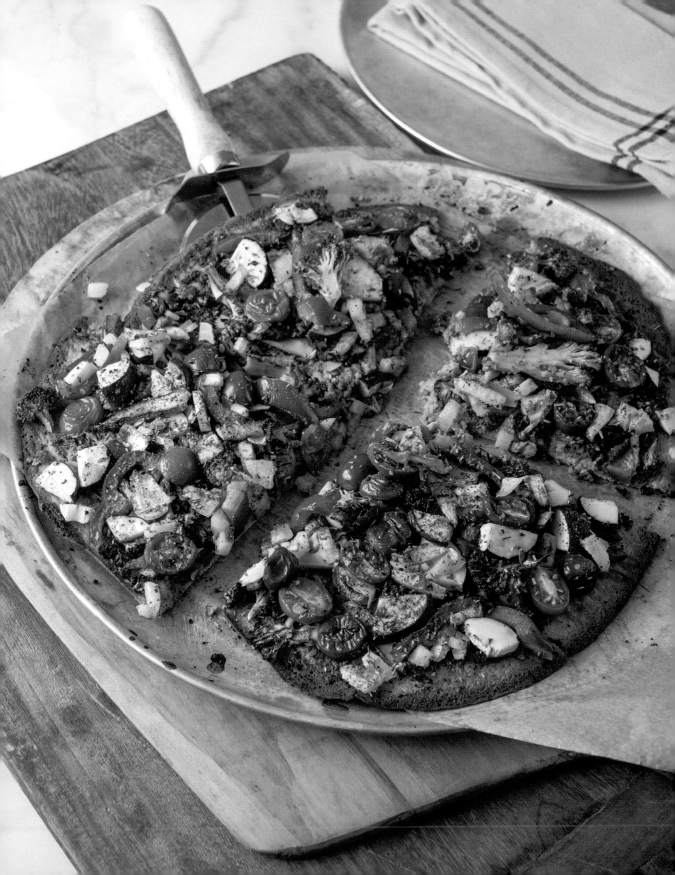

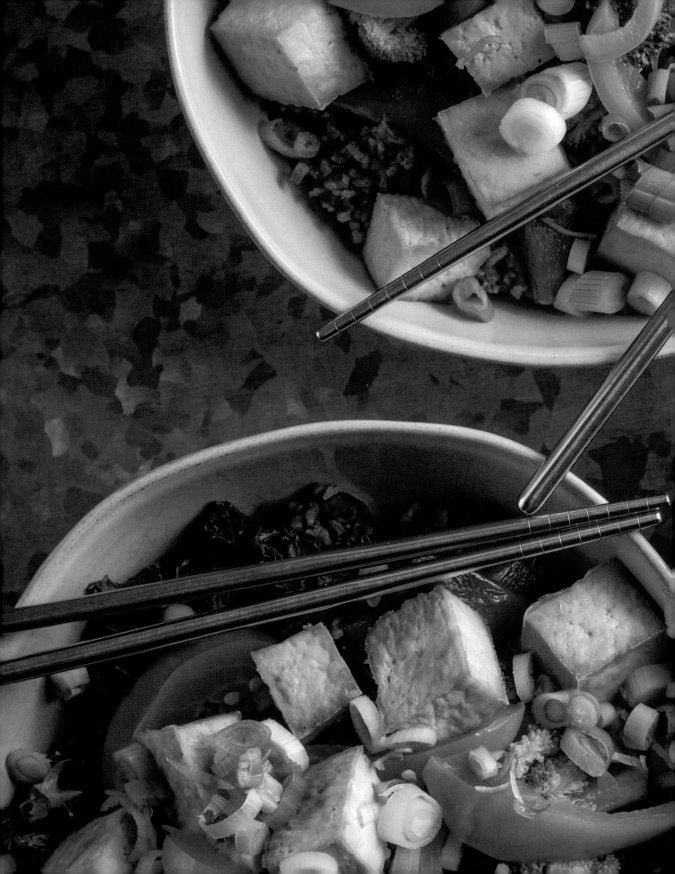

VEGGIE BOWLS

Rice, beans, avocado, salsa, cilantro, fresh mango … interested? Veggie bowls are a quick way to whip up a hearty and delicious plant-based meal with your pantry staples. Just pile your favorites into a bowl and enjoy.

We've purposely kept the preparations pared down to make shopping for and preparing these a breeze. We've included four of our favorite combinations to get you started, but feel free to use your creativity (and your leftovers) to make your own perfect bowl.

PRO TIP: Keep a selection of cooked beans, seasoned veggies, and grains like rice or quinoa in the fridge. Simply prepare these ingredients when you have a few extra minutes on the weekend, and they'll be ready to warm up and bowl when you are.

PARADISE BOWL

Yield: 1 bowl | *Serves 1*

½ cup black rice, cooked according to the package instructions

½ cup Roasted Plantains (page 167)

½ cup Cumin Black Beans (page 162)

¼ cup Apple Cider Onions (page 165)

½ cup Pineapple Pico (page 168)

¼ cup Corn Guacamole (page 167)

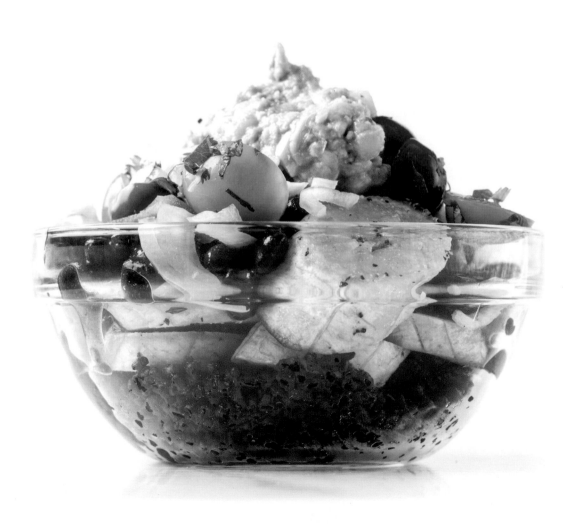

CURRY BOWL

Yield: 1 bowl | *Serves 1*

½ cup red or brown rice, cooked according to the package instructions

½ cup Curried Cauliflower (page 165)

¼ cup Apple Cider Onions (page 165)

¼ cup Shake & Bake Chickpeas (page 220)

¼ cup fresh mango

¼ cup Apple-Ginger Kimchi (page 200)

Cilantro, to garnish

Coconut aminos, lightly drizzled (optional)

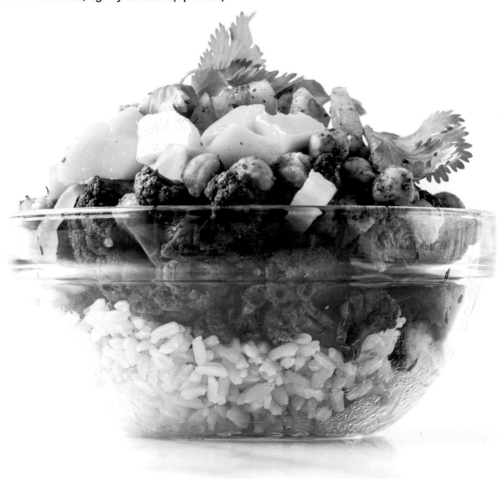

FIESTA BOWL

Yield: 1 bowl | *Serves 1*

½ cup red or brown rice, cooked according to the package instructions

½ cup Cumin Black Beans (page 162)

½ cup Cinnamon Sweet Potatoes (page 164)

½ cup Maple Mustard Cabbage (page 163)

½ cup Chinese Five-Spice Tofu (page 163)

¼ cup Super-Fresh Salsa (page 195)

¼ cup Corn Guacamole (page 167)

Sliced sweet peppers, to garnish

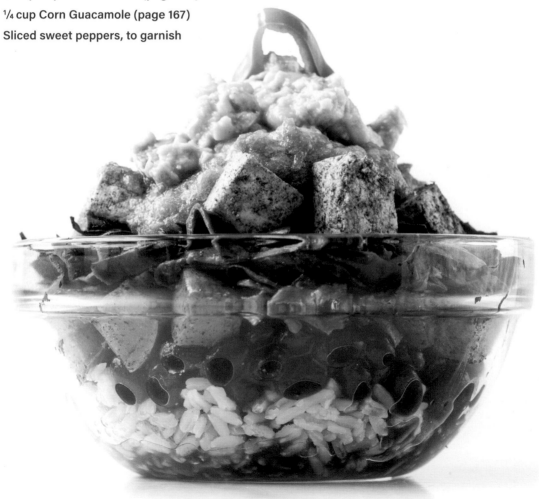

PEANUT BOWL

Yield: 1 bowl | *Serves 1*

½ cup black or red rice, cooked according to the package instructions

¼ cup edamame

½ cup sliced sweet peppers

½ cup Balsamic Broccoli (page 164)

½ cup Chinese Five-Spice Tofu (page 163)

¼ cup Spicy Nut Butter Sauce (page 203)

Cilantro, to garnish

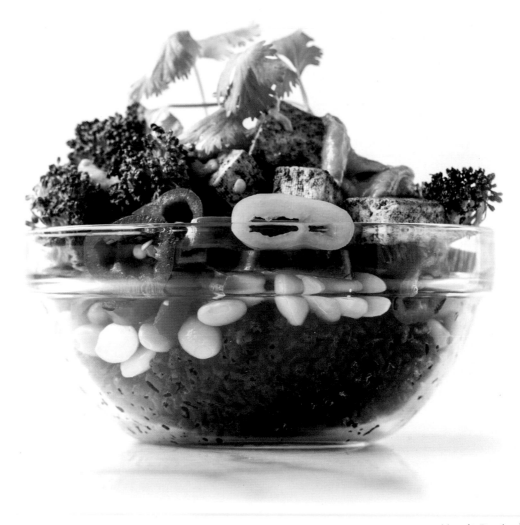

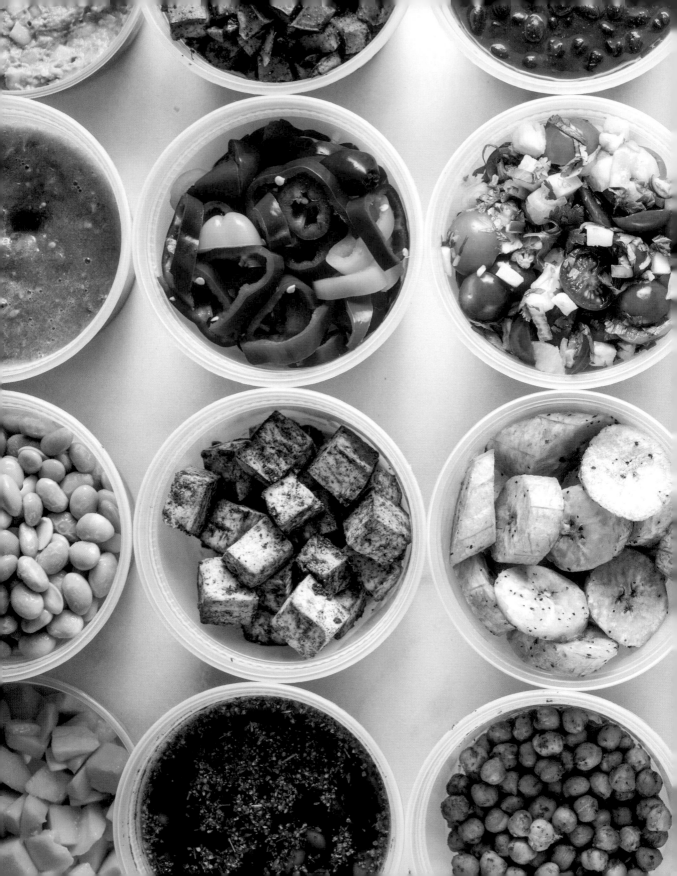

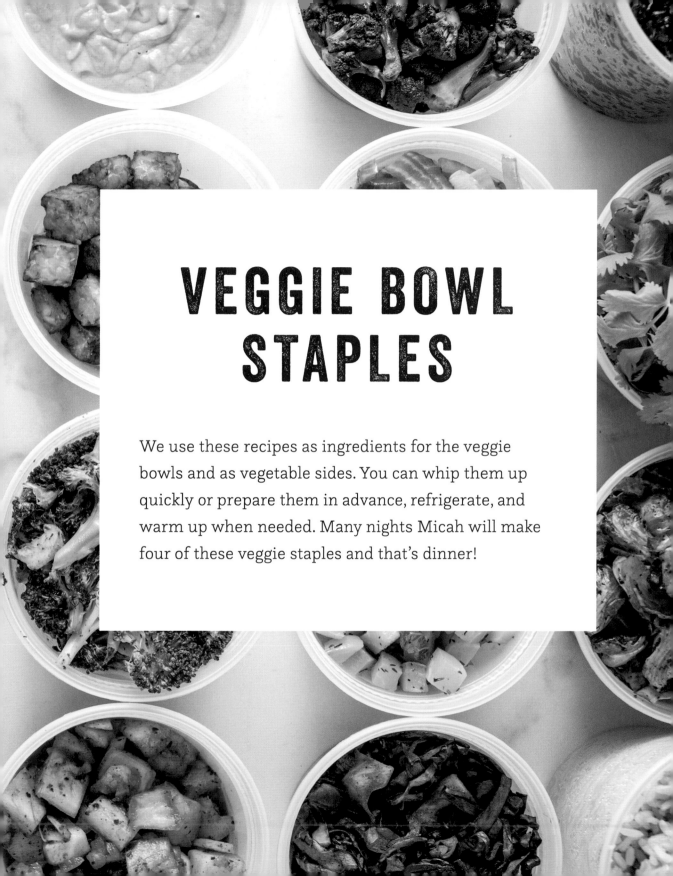

VEGGIE BOWL STAPLES

We use these recipes as ingredients for the veggie bowls and as vegetable sides. You can whip them up quickly or prepare them in advance, refrigerate, and warm up when needed. Many nights Micah will make four of these veggie staples and that's dinner!

RED, BLACK, OR BROWN RICE

Yield: 1 quart | *Serves 8*

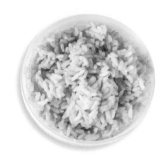

4 cups prepared rice of your choice cooked according to the package instructions

CUMIN BLACK BEANS

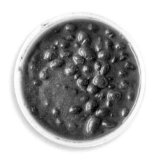

Yield: 3 cups | *Serves 6*

Two 15.5-ounce cans black beans with liquid, or 3 cups cooked black beans with up to 12 ounces water or vegetable broth

2 teaspoons cumin

1 teaspoon ground coriander

½ teaspoon sea salt

Place all the ingredients in a small saucepan. Set over medium heat and cook until heated through.

PAPRIKA PINTO BEANS

Yield: 3 cups | *Serves 6*

Two 15.5-ounce cans pinto beans with liquid, or 3 cups cooked pinto beans with up to 12 ounces water or vegetable broth

2 teaspoons dried oregano

½ teaspoon sea salt

1 tablespoon sweet paprika

Heat the beans with their liquid, along with the oregano, paprika, and salt in a small saucepan over medium heat.

SHAKE & BAKE CHICKPEAS

Yield: 1 cups | *Serves 4*

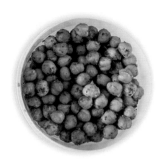

See Shake & Bake Chickpeas recipe on page 220.

CHINESE FIVE-SPICE TOFU

Yield: 2 cups | *Serves 4*

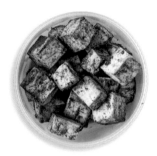

One 14-ounce package extra-firm tofu, drained and cubed

1 teaspoon Chinese five-spice powder

1 tablespoon coconut aminos

1. Preheat your oven to 400°F.

2. Toss the tofu, Chinese five-spice, and coconut aminos in a large mixing bowl until the tofu is well coated.

3. Spread the mixture, along with any liquid in the bowl, on a parchment-lined baking sheet. Bake for 20 minutes.

MAPLE MUSTARD CABBAGE

Yield: 2 cups | *Serves 4*

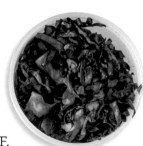

4 cups shredded red or purple cabbage (from about ½ of a medium head)

1 tablespoon spicy mustard

1 teaspoon maple syrup

1. Preheat your oven to 400°F.

2. Toss all the ingredients in a large mixing bowl until the cabbage is well coated.

3. Spread the mixture, along with any liquid in the bowl, on a parchment-lined baking sheet. Bake for 20 minutes.

CINNAMON SWEET POTATOES

Yield: 3 cups | *Serves 6*

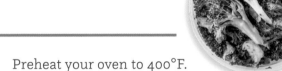

2 large sweet potatoes, cubed (about 4 cups)

1 to 2 teaspoons extra-virgin olive oil

½ teaspoon cinnamon

½ teaspoon black pepper

¼ teaspoon sea salt

1. Preheat your oven to 400°F.

2. Toss all the ingredients in a large mixing bowl until the sweet potatoes are well coated.

3. Spread the mixture, along with any liquid in the bowl, on a parchment-lined baking sheet. Bake for 20 minutes.

BALSAMIC BROCCOLI

Yield: 2½ cups | *Serves 6*

1 large broccoli crown, broken into florets (about 4 cups)

1 teaspoon extra-virgin olive oil

1 teaspoon balsamic vinegar

2 teaspoons Italian seasoning

¼ teaspoon sea salt

1. Preheat your oven to 400°F.

2. Toss all the ingredients in a large mixing bowl until the broccoli is well coated.

3. Spread the mixture, along with any liquid in the bowl, on a parchment-lined baking sheet. Bake for 20 minutes.

CURRIED CAULIFLOWER

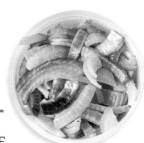

Yield: 2 ½ cups | *Serves 6*

1 small head of cauliflower
(about 4 cups)

1 teaspoon extra-virgin
olive oil

2 teaspoons curry powder
or Anticancer Sprinkle
(page 19)

1. Preheat your oven to 400°F.

2. Toss all the ingredients in a large mixing bowl
   until the cauliflower is well coated.

3. Spread the mixture, along with any liquid in the
   bowl, on a parchment-lined baking sheet. Bake
   for 20 minutes.

APPLE CIDER ONIONS

Yield: 2 cups | *Serves 8*

1 large red onion, thinly sliced
into half-moons (about 4 cups)

1 teaspoon sesame oil

1 teaspoon coconut aminos

1 tablespoon apple cider
vinegar

1. Preheat your oven to 400°F.

2. Toss all the ingredients in a large mixing bowl
   until the onions are well coated.

3. Spread the mixture, along with any liquid in the
   bowl, on a parchment-lined baking sheet. Bake
   for 20 minutes.

SAVORY BRUSSELS SPROUTS

Yield: 3 cups | *Serves 6*

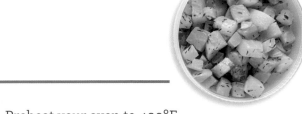

1 pound Brussels sprouts, trimmed and quartered

1 to 2 teaspoons toasted sesame oil

1 teaspoon sweet paprika

¼ teaspoon sea salt

¼ teaspoon black pepper

1. Preheat your oven to 400°F.

2. Toss all the ingredients in a large mixing bowl until the Brussels sprouts are well coated.

3. Spread the mixture, along with any liquid in the bowl, on a parchment-lined baking sheet. Bake for 20 minutes.

SWEET BEETS

Yield: 2 to 3 cups | *Serves 6*

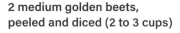

2 medium golden beets, peeled and diced (2 to 3 cups)

1 teaspoon extra-virgin olive oil

1 teaspoon apple cider vinegar

½ teaspoon dried thyme

¼ teaspoon sea salt

1. Preheat your oven to 400°F.

2. Toss all the ingredients in a large mixing bowl until the beets are well coated.

3. Spread the mixture, along with any liquid in the bowl, on a parchment-lined baking sheet. Bake for 20 minutes.

ROASTED PLANTAINS

Yield: 3 cups | *Serves 6*

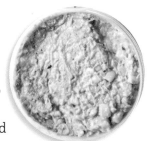

2 medium-size ripe plantains, peeled and sliced

1 tablespoon coconut oil or extra-virgin olive oil

Juice of 1 lime

⅛ teaspoon sea salt

1. Preheat your oven to 400°F.

2. Toss all the ingredients in a large mixing bowl until the plantains are well coated.

3. Spread the mixture, along with any liquid in the bowl, on a parchment-lined baking sheet. Bake for 20 minutes.

NOTE: Look for plantains that don't have any green on them. You want the peel to look yellow and black like an overripe banana.

PRO TIP: You can use slightly underripe bananas in place of the plantains in this recipe. Bananas are easier to find and always delicious.

CORN GUACAMOLE

2 cups guacamole or Guac of Ages (page 192)

1 cup corn kernels, cooked

Combine the guacamole and corn in a large mixing bowl.

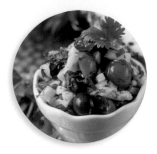

PINEAPPLE PICO

Yield: 3 cups | *Serves 6*

1 cup diced pineapple

1 pint cherry tomatoes, halved

Juice of 1 lime

1 medium shallot, diced

1 medium jalapeño, sliced

½ cup cilantro

¼ teaspoon sea salt

Toss all the ingredients in a large mixing bowl until well mixed.

SPICY NUT BUTTER SAUCE

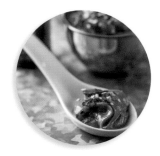

See Spicy Nut Butter Sauce recipe on page 203.

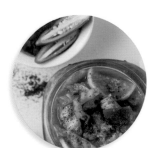

APPLE-GINGER KIMCHI

See Apple-Ginger Kimchi recipe on page 200.

SUPER-FRESH SALSA

See Super-Fresh Salsa recipe on page 195.

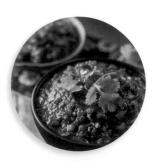

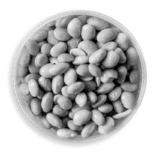

EDAMAME

One 8-ounce package frozen edamame, cooked according to the package instructions

FRESH CILANTRO

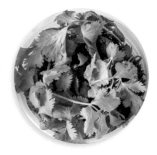

1 medium bunch cilantro, trimmed

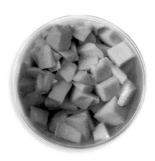

FRESH MANGO

2 medium Champagne mangoes, peeled, seeded, and diced

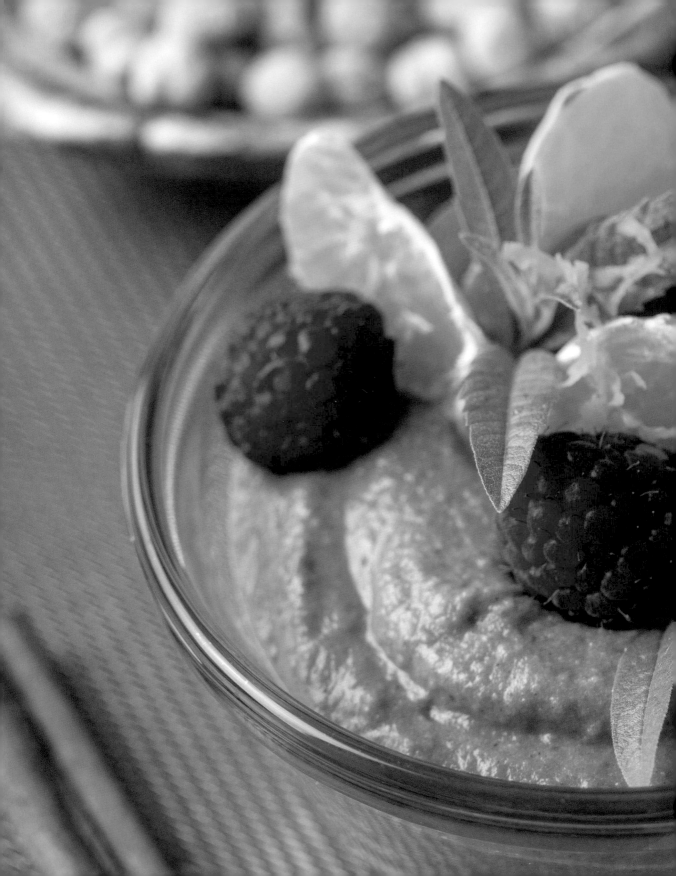

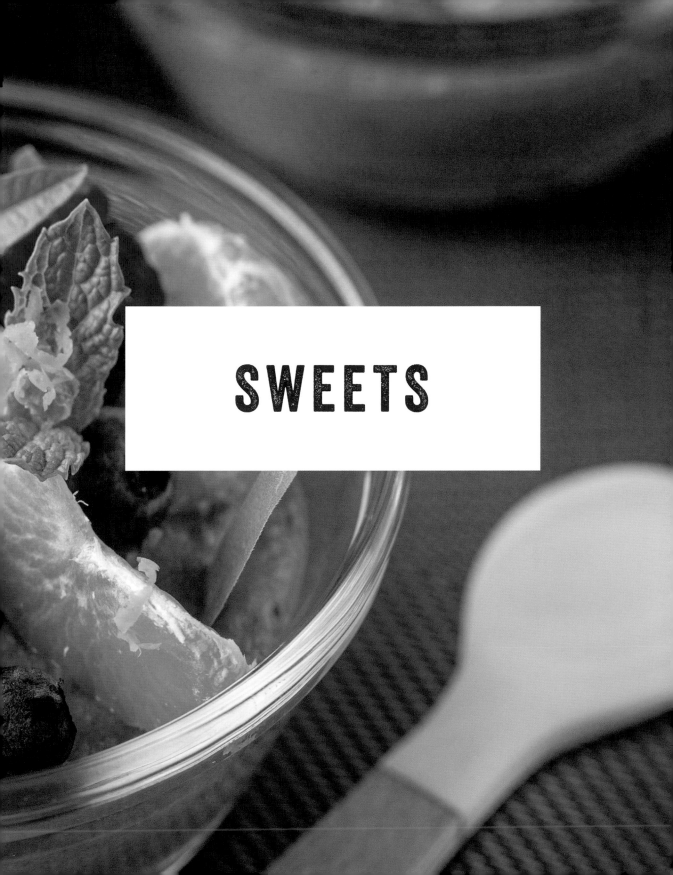

SWEETS

MANGO FORBIDDEN RICE
with Maple Ginger Lime Drizzle

Rice paired with fruit is a dessert staple in many parts of Asia. This Thai-inspired dessert combines melt-in-your-mouth sweet mango with "superantioxidant" black rice and our spectacular Maple Ginger Lime Drizzle.

Yield: 4 cups | *Serves 4*

2 cups black rice

Juice of 2 limes
(about ¼ cup)

1 teaspoon grated fresh
ginger

2 tablespoons maple syrup,
plus more for drizzling

⅛ teaspoon cayenne
pepper

⅛ teaspoon sea salt

3 medium mangoes, diced

1. Cook the rice according to the package directions and keep warm.

2. Whisk the lime juice, ginger, maple syrup, cayenne pepper, and salt in a medium bowl.

3. Serve ½ cup of rice topped with diced mango and Maple Ginger Lime Drizzle.

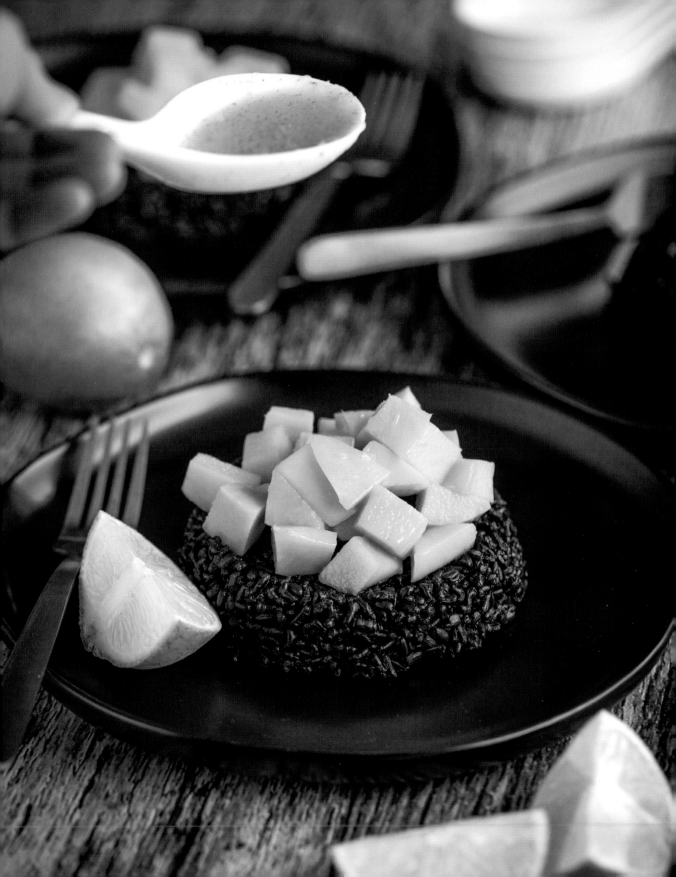

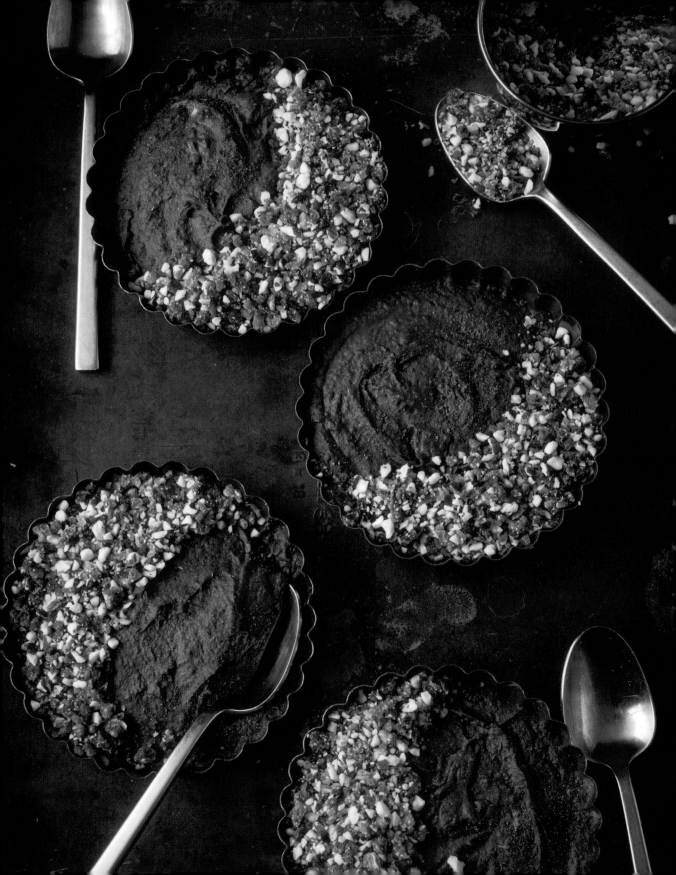

PURPLE SWEET POTATO PIES
with Almond Date Crumble

We tossed out all the junk in traditional sweet potato pie—white flour, white sugar, butter, and hours of work—and created a super-nutritious dessert that's a cinch to prepare.

Yield: 1 quart | *Serves 4*

2 medium purple sweet potatoes

½ cup pitted dates

½ cup whole almonds

¼ cup creamy almond butter

1 teaspoon pumpkin pie spice

½ cup apple juice

1 tablespoon maple syrup

1 teaspoon vanilla extract

¼ teaspoon sea salt

1. Preheat your oven to 350°F.

2. Bake the sweet potatoes on a baking sheet for 45 minutes.

3. Once the potatoes are cool enough to handle, peel the skin.

4. Pulse the dates and almonds in the work bowl of a food processor until crumbled to the size of a dried lentil. Remove the crumble from the processor and set aside.

5. Place the baked sweet potatoes, almond butter, pumpkin pie spice, apple juice, maple syrup, vanilla, and salt in the work bowl of a food processor and blend until just smooth.

6. Divide the mixture into four small, wide, shallow bowls, and top with the almond and date crumble.

NOTE: Purple sweet potatoes have higher levels of cancer-fighting anthocyanins, but if you can't find purple ones, regular sweet potatoes will definitely do the trick.

NO-BAKE PEANUT CACAO CUPS

Adults love them. Kids love them. Everyone loves them. Our No-Bake Peanut Cacao Cups are a fantastic sweet treat for dessert with a glass of your favorite nut milk.

Yield: 8 cups | *Serves 8*

1 cup peanuts, plus
¼ cup chopped peanuts
for topping

1 cup pitted dates

¼ cup cacao or cocoa
powder

1 teaspoon vanilla extract

¼ cup smooth peanut
butter (almond and cashew
butter are great too)

Maple Cacao Topping
(recipe follows)

1. Pulse the peanuts, dates, cacao powder, and vanilla in the work bowl of a food processor until everything is the size of grains of rice.

2. Add the peanut butter and pulse to combine until smooth but grainy.

3. Using a muffin tin, firmly press ¼ cup of the mixture into the bottom of 1 cup. Repeat until all the mixture is used.

4. Distribute the Maple Cacao topping evenly among the cups and sprinkle the tops with chopped peanuts.

5. Refrigerate for 1 hour before removing from the muffin tin.

PRO TIP: Double the recipe and keep a batch in the freezer for later. These go fast!

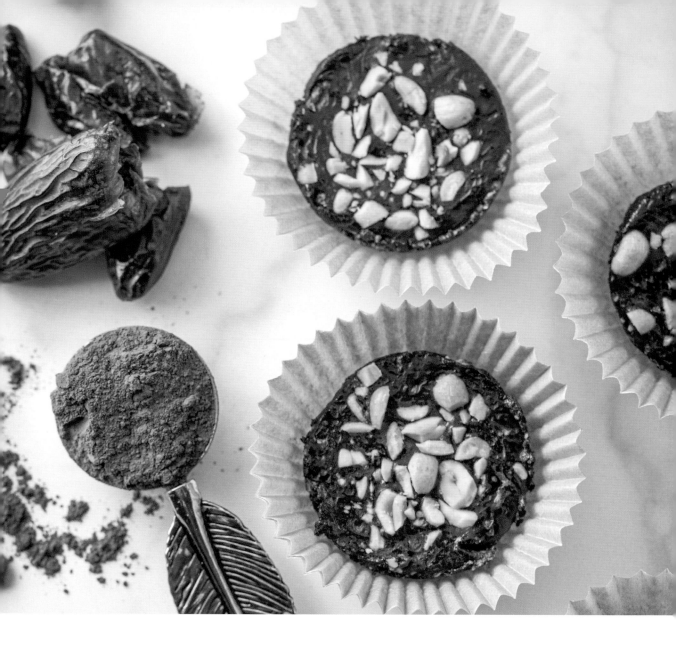

MAPLE CACAO TOPPING

2 tablespoons cacao powder

2 tablespoons maple syrup

2 tablespoons coconut oil

Whisk all the ingredients in a small mixing bowl until smooth.

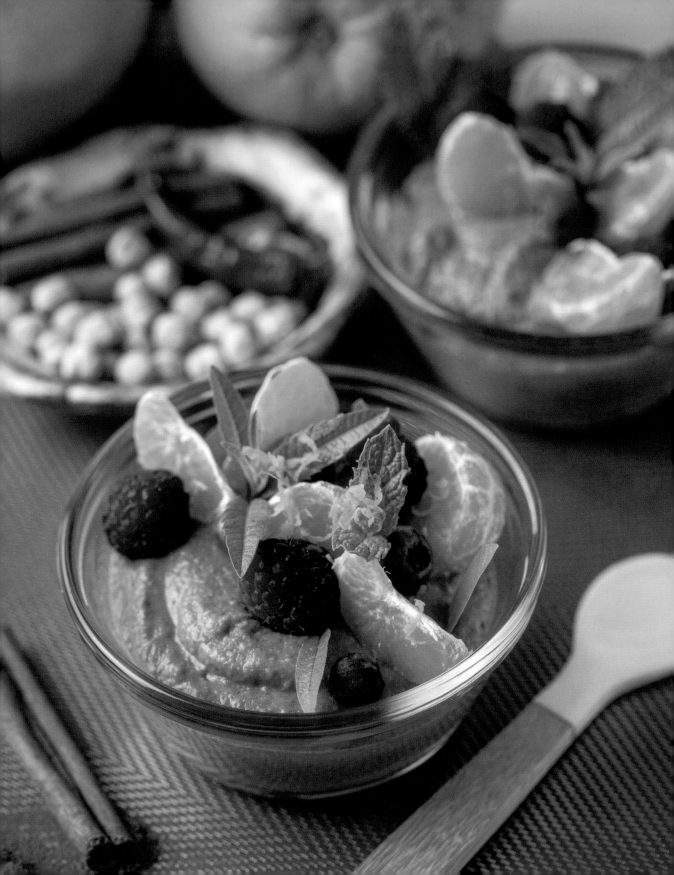

MEXICAN CHOCOLATE HUMMUS

If you love chocolate and you love hummus, you're going to flip for our south of the border–inspired Mexican Chocolate Hummus spiced with cayenne and orange zest and sweetened with maple syrup. This is guaranteed to score you some points with your highfalutin foodie friends. Dip sliced apples or your favorite fresh fruit in it and enjoy!

Yield: 2 1/2 cups | *Serves 4*

½ cup pitted dates, soaked in hot water for 30 minutes and drained

One 15-ounce can chickpeas, drained, or 1½ cups cooked chickpeas

Zest and juice of 1 medium orange (about ⅓ cup juice)

1 teaspoon cocoa powder

¼ teaspoon cinnamon

⅛ teaspoon salt

2 tablespoons tahini

2 tablespoons maple syrup

⅛ teaspoon cayenne pepper (optional)

1 cup of your favorite fresh fruit, mint leaves, and lemon verbena, to garnish

1. Blend the dates, chickpeas, orange zest and juice, cocoa powder, cinnamon, salt, tahini, maple syrup, and cayenne pepper, if using, in the work bowl of a food processor until very smooth.

2. Divide the mixture into 4 small bowls, and garnish with fruit, mint leaves, and lemon verbena. Chill in the fridge until ready to serve.

NOTE: Dates do not blend as easily as chickpeas, which is why we soak them first. Be patient and allow your food processor to do the work. You'll notice the dates jumping around in the work bowl at first. This is normal.

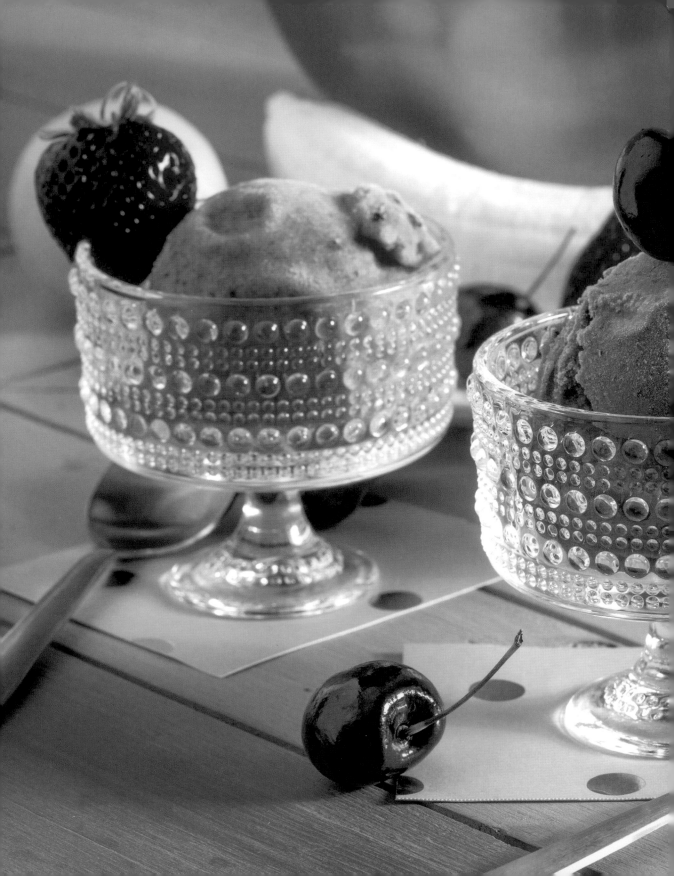

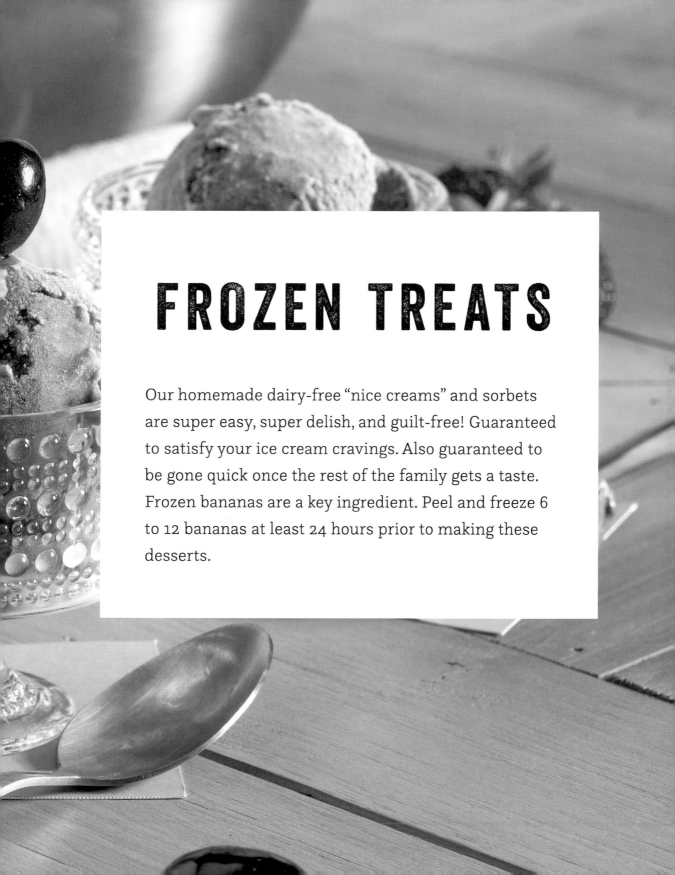

FROZEN TREATS

Our homemade dairy-free "nice creams" and sorbets are super easy, super delish, and guilt-free! Guaranteed to satisfy your ice cream cravings. Also guaranteed to be gone quick once the rest of the family gets a taste. Frozen bananas are a key ingredient. Peel and freeze 6 to 12 bananas at least 24 hours prior to making these desserts.

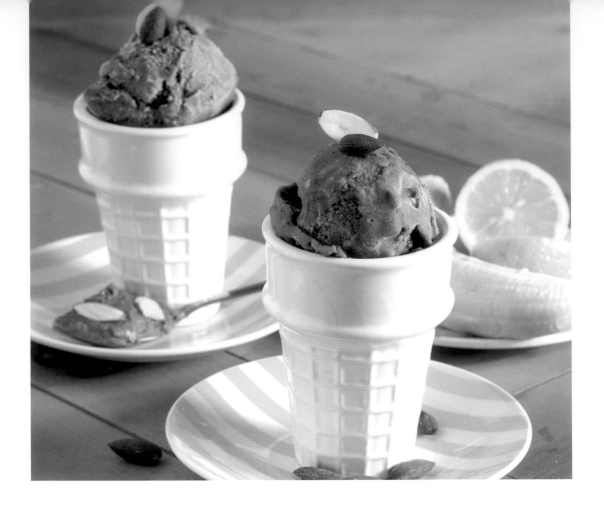

CACAO ALMOND BANANA NICE CREAM

Yield: 2 cups | *Serves 4*

Juice of 1 lemon

1 teaspoon vanilla extract

¼ cup almond milk

2 teaspoons cacao powder or cocoa powder

3 frozen ripe bananas, peeled and sliced into 6 pieces each

¼ cup almond butter

1. Gently blend the lemon juice, vanilla extract, almond milk, and cacao powder in a food processor or high-powered blender. Then add the bananas and blend all the ingredients together until smooth.

2. Add the almond butter and pulse 3 to 4 times to swirl the almond butter into the mix. Serve immediately or freeze in an airtight container for up to 30 days.

STRAWBERRY-LEMON SORBET

Yield: 2 cups | *Serves 4*

2 frozen ripe bananas, peeled and sliced into 6 pieces each

1 cup strawberries, cut in half

¼ cup almond milk

Juice of 1 lemon

1 teaspoon vanilla extract

Blend all the ingredients together in a food processor or high-powered blender until smooth. Serve immediately or freeze in an airtight container for up to 30 days.

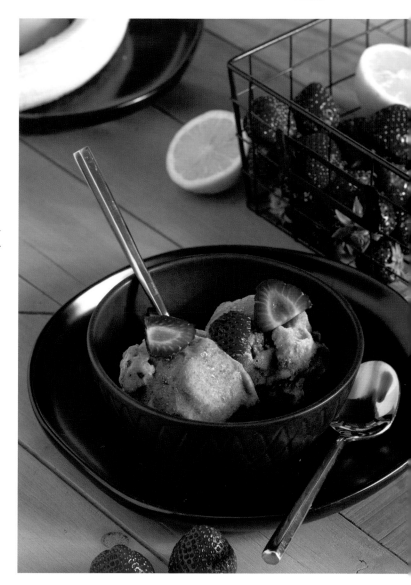

CHERRY CASHEW CACAO NICE CREAM

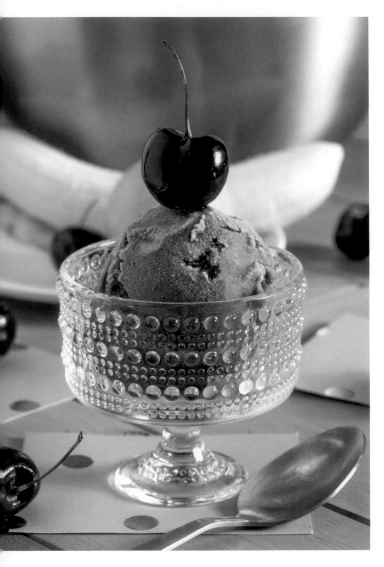

¼ cup cashew milk
or almond milk

Juice of 1 lemon

1 teaspoon vanilla extract

2 teaspoons cacao powder or
cocoa powder

2 frozen ripe bananas, peeled
and sliced into 6 pieces each

1 cup frozen cherries or fresh
pitted cherries

Gently blend the cashew milk, lemon juice, vanilla extract, and cacao powder in a food processor or high-powered blender. Then add the bananas and cherries and blend until smooth. Serve immediately or freeze in an airtight container for up to 30 days.

PRO TIP: For a richer, creamier version, add ¼ cup of cashew butter and swirl it into the mix with 3 to 4 pulses after all the other ingredients have been blended.

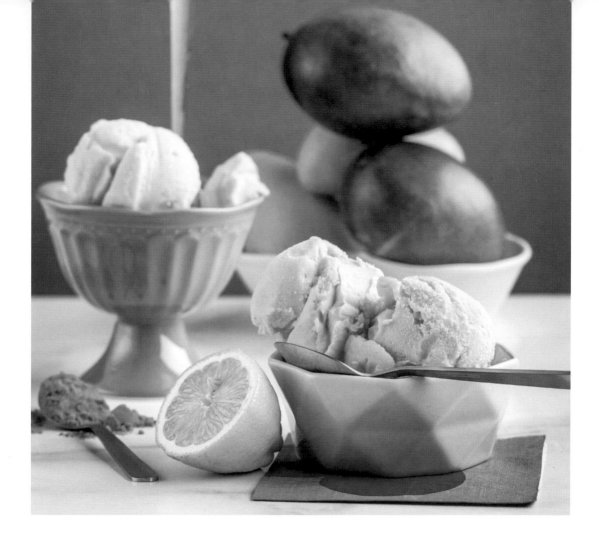

MANGO TURMERIC TART SORBET

Juice of 1 lemon

1 teaspoon vanilla extract

¼ cup cashew or almond milk

¼ teaspoon turmeric powder

2 frozen ripe bananas, peeled and sliced into 6 pieces each

1 cup frozen mango chunks

Gently blend the lemon juice, vanilla extract, nut milk, and turmeric powder in a food processor or high-powered blender. Then add the bananas and mango and blend until smooth. Serve immediately or freeze in an airtight container for up to 30 days.

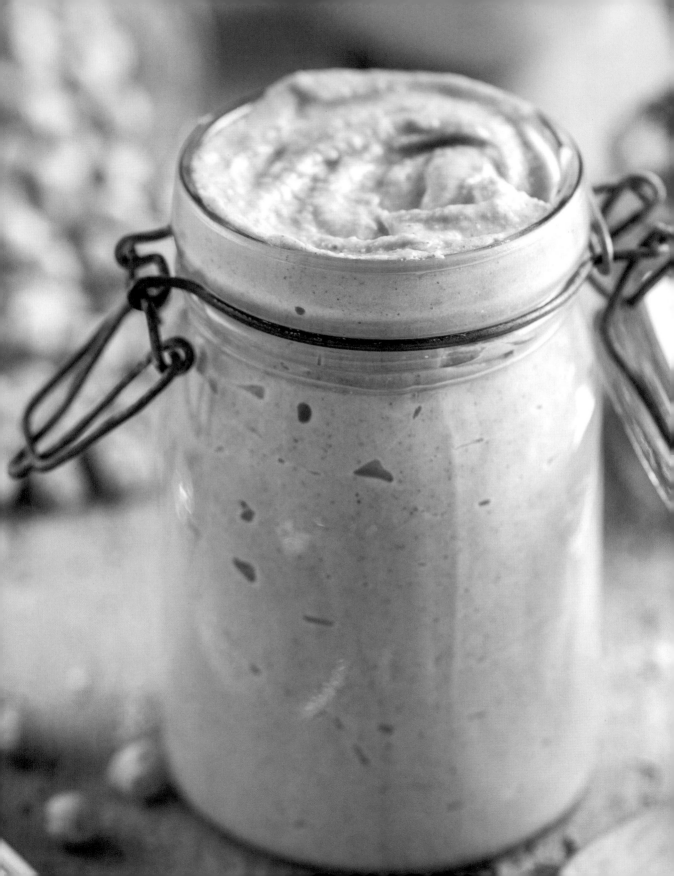

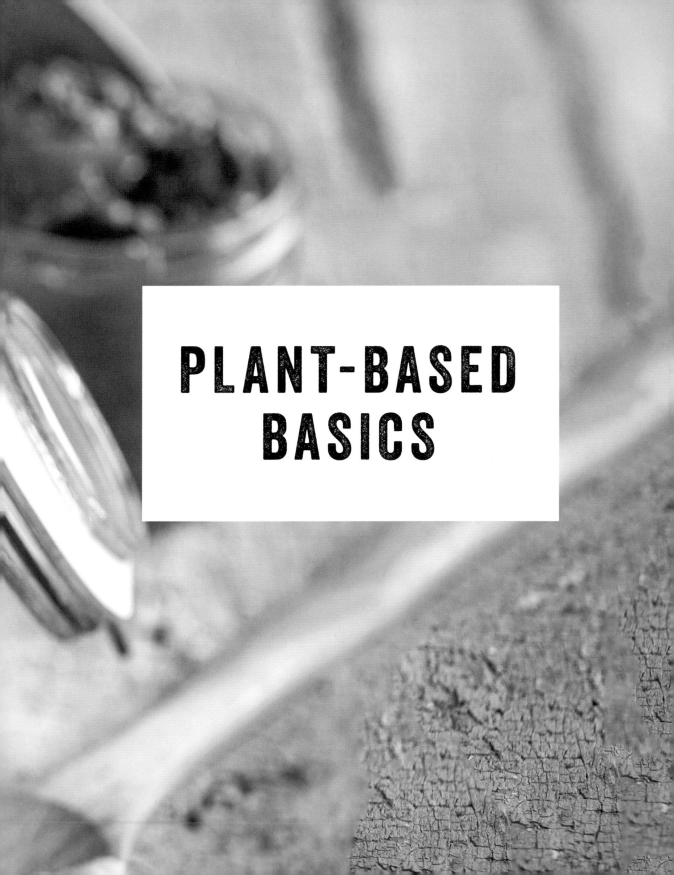

PLANT-BASED BASICS

BROCCOLI SPROUT PESTO

It's hard to improve on pesto, but we did it . . . with broccoli sprouts! Broccoli sprouts contain the highest concentrations of sulforaphane and indole-3-carbinol, two compounds that improve detoxification and immune function. Broccoli sprouts give pesto a peppery kick and anticancer superpowers. Perfect for dips, pizza, pasta, and sandwich spreads. Enjoy!

Yield: 1¹/₂ cups | *Serves 4 to 6*

4 ounces broccoli sprouts

2 ounces fresh basil leaves, large stems discarded

¹/₃ cup pine nuts, toasted

1 tablespoon nutritional yeast

¹/₂ teaspoon sea salt

¹/₂ teaspoon black pepper

Zest and juice of 1 medium lemon

¹/₂ teaspoon maple syrup

2 tablespoons extra-virgin olive oil

1. Blend the broccoli sprouts, basil leaves, pine nuts, nutritional yeast, salt, pepper, lemon zest and juice, and maple syrup in the work bowl of your food processor while drizzling in the olive oil in a light and steady stream.

2. Scrape the sides down using a soft spatula and blend the mixture until smooth.

One cup of broccoli sprouts has roughly 25 times more of the anticancer supernutrient sulforaphane than a cup of mature broccoli.

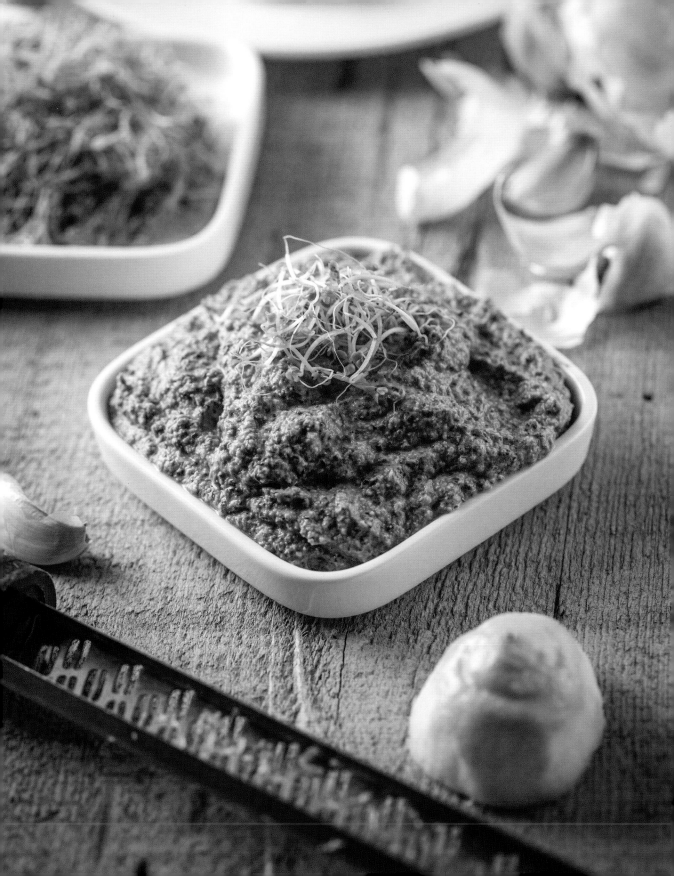

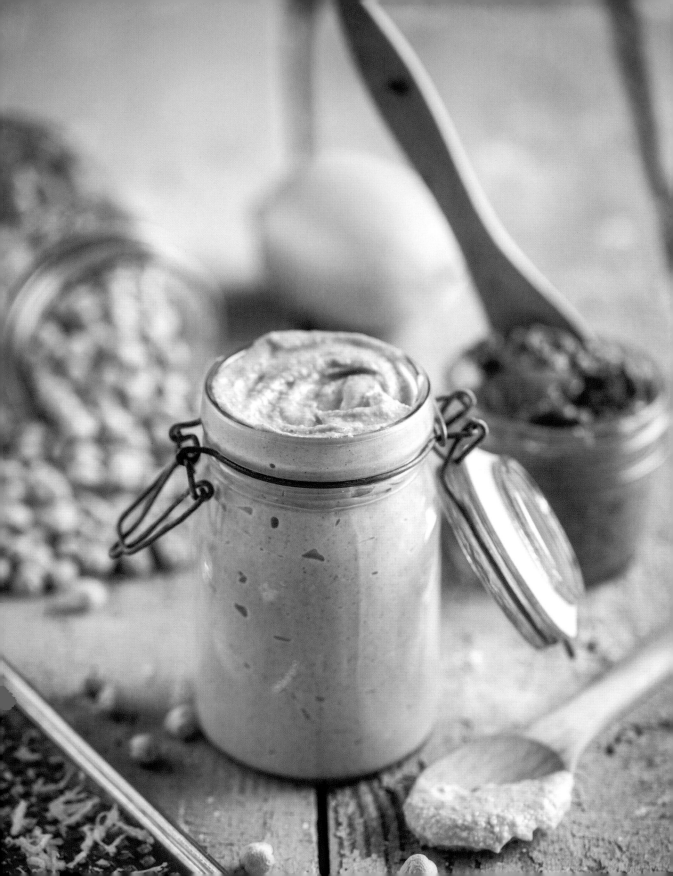

LEMONY ALMOND HUMMUS

Our hummus with chickpeas, lemon, and almond butter is delicious, oil-free, and super versatile. Use it as a sandwich spread or as a veggie dip. It is also the base of our fabulous Jalapeño Strawberry Avocado Toast (page 48).

Yield: 1½ cups | *Serves 4 to 6*

One 15-ounce can chickpeas, drained and rinsed

3 tablespoons water

¼ cup smooth almond butter

Zest and juice of 1 medium lemon

½ teaspoon sea salt

2 tablespoons hemp hearts

Blend all the ingredients in the work bowl of a food processor or in a blender until smooth.

GUAC OF AGES

Avocados are a wonderful source of healthy fat and fiber, and guacamole makes nearly every dish infinitely better. Our Guac of Ages has a touch of maple syrup to give a hint of sweetness to this yummy classic. For those about to guac . . . we salute you!

Yield: 2 ¼ cups | *Serves 4*

4 medium avocados, peeled and pits removed

¼ cup minced red onion (from about ¼ of a medium onion)

Juice from 1 to 2 medium limes (about 1 tablespoon)

½ teaspoon maple syrup

½ teaspoon sea salt

½ teaspoon black pepper

½ to 1 small garlic clove, minced

Use a fork to mash together all the ingredients in a medium bowl, leaving some avocado chunks for texture. Store in the fridge until ready to use.

PRO TIP: Make guacamole within 30 minutes of serving so it doesn't brown.

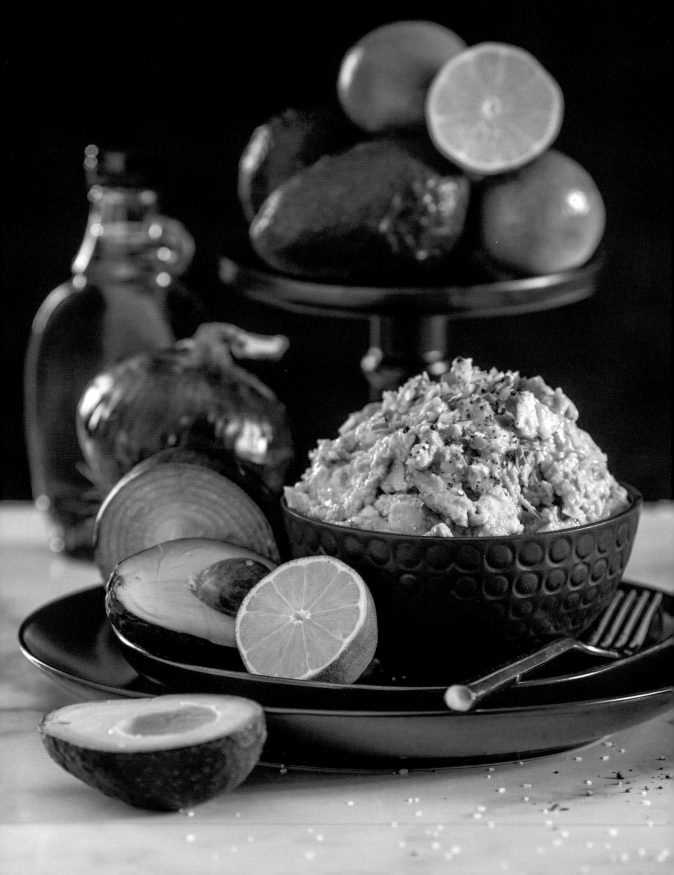

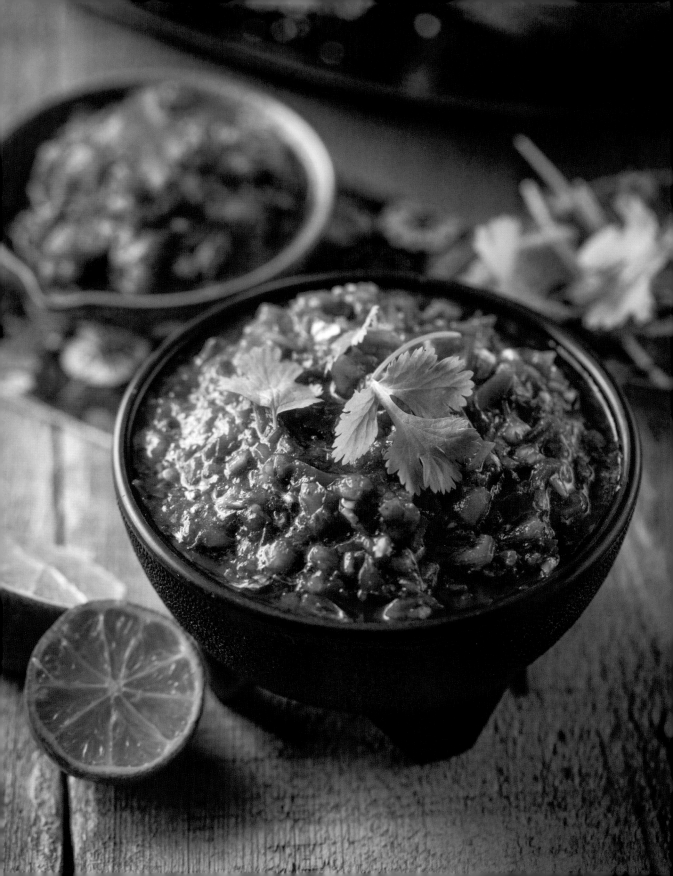

SUPER-FRESH SALSA

Fresh tomatoes, garlic, jalapeño, lime, and cilantro … nothing beats homemade salsa. Here's how we make it at our house.

Yield: 3 cups | *Serves 4 to 6*

---

2 garlic cloves, peeled

1 large jalapeño, stem and seeds removed

2 tablespoons tomato paste

Juice of 2 limes

1 cup loose-packed cilantro leaves

5 to 6 large Roma tomatoes, roughly chopped (about 4 cups)

½ teaspoon sea salt

Blend all the ingredients in the work bowl of a food processor with quick pulses until your desired consistency is reached.

NO HARM PARM

Here's an easy "cheesy" topping with no dairy necessary. Just mix a few *Beat Cancer Kitchen* pantry staples together, and you have a tasty topping for pastas, salads, and veggies. Nutritional yeast is a great source of vitamin B_{12} and beta-glucans. The hemp hearts amp it up with protein, omega-3 and omega-6 fats, fiber, magnesium, and iron.

Yield: 1 cup

½ cup hemp hearts

½ cup nutritional yeast

1 teaspoon sea salt, crushed

⅛ teaspoon granulated garlic

Zest of 1 medium lemon

Shake all the ingredients together in a sealed container such as a Mason jar until well combined. Use anywhere you'd use Parmesan cheese.

Nutritional yeast contains beta-glucan, an immunomodulatory compound that enhances your body's defenses against infections and cancer.[70] Beta-glucans have been shown to increase immune function, specifically monocyte and natural killer cell activity against cancer.[71] In one study, breast cancer patients who were given a small amount of beta-glucan daily—the equivalent of 1/16 teaspoon of nutritional yeast—had a 50 percent increase in monocytes in their bloodstream after just two weeks.[72]

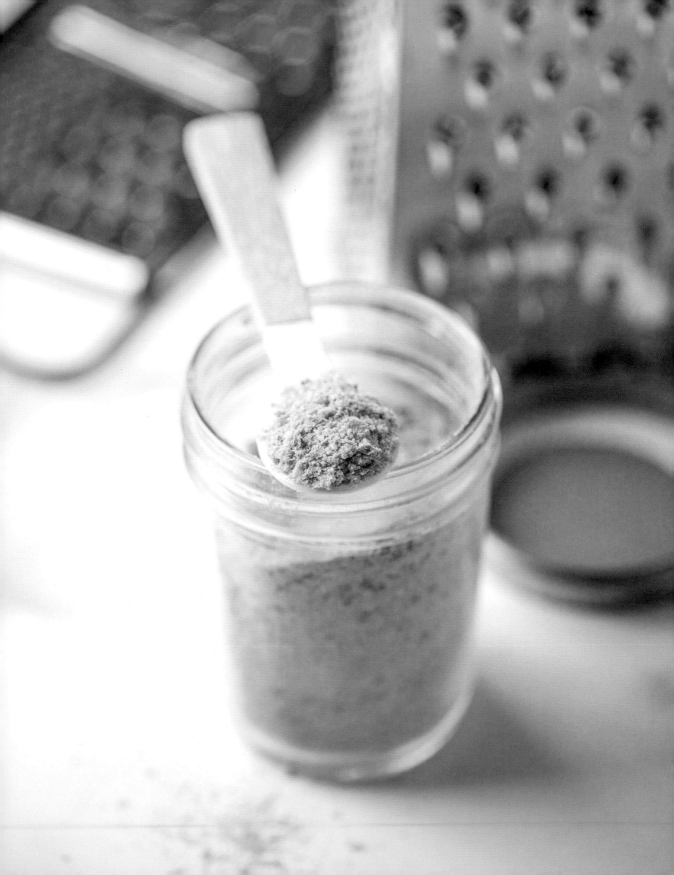

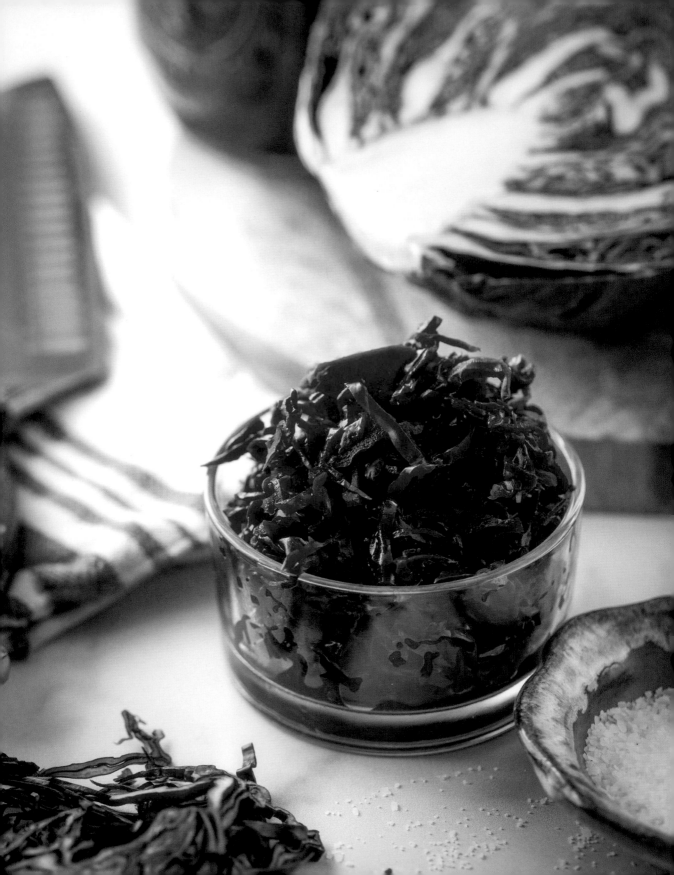

RUBY KRAUT

Sauerkraut is a delicious fermented food made from cabbage, water, and salt. Using red or purple cabbage instead of green yields a vibrant, colorful sauerkraut with higher levels of cancer-fighting anthocyanins. Sauerkraut serves as a tasty side or topping to make sandwiches, salads, and veggie bowls pop.

Yield: 4 cups

6 cups finely shredded purple cabbage

1 tablespoon sea salt

1. Throw a handful of shredded cabbage and a pinch of salt into a large bowl. Repeat until all the cabbage and salt have been used.

2. Cover the bowl and allow the cabbage to sit on the kitchen counter for 1 hour.

3. Using clean hands, knead the cabbage in the bowl and squeeze it in your fists. Do not throw out the liquid that is extracted.

4. Pack the cabbage into a quart-size Mason jar, pushing it to the bottom, and add the liquid from the bowl on top. Add enough water (a few tablespoons) as needed to just cover the cabbage. Leave about an inch of headspace as the cabbage will expand when it comes alive and begins to bubble.

5. Leave the jar lid loose and the jar on the countertop for 24 to 48 hours, or until the desired tanginess is achieved. Then it's ready to eat.

6. Tighten the lid and store in the fridge for up to a month.

Red or purple cabbage is one of the most economically healthy foods. It is one of the highest-antioxidant and lowest-priced plant foods next to broccoli sprouts.[73]

APPLE-GINGER KIMCHI

Kimchi, a spicy Korean version of sauerkraut, is considered one of the world's healthiest foods due to its immune-boosting, anti-inflammatory, anticancer, and beneficial bacterial content. Our Apple-Ginger Kimchi adds a sweet, savory, spicy goodness to the Giant Cancer-Fighting Salad, a rice bowl, or any dish you want to jazz up.

Yield: 6 cups

1 medium sweet apple, such as Fuji, Gala, or Pink Lady

1-inch piece of fresh ginger

1 medium jalapeño, seeded and stem removed

6 medium garlic cloves, peeled

2 tablespoons paprika

1 tablespoon coconut aminos

¼ cup water

6 to 8 cups shredded napa cabbage, rinsed and drained

1 tablespoon sea salt

3 medium green onions, sliced

1 cup sliced radishes

1. Using the work bowl of a food processor, blend the whole apple, ginger, jalapeño, garlic, paprika, coconut aminos, and water into a paste. Set aside.

2. Place a handful of cabbage in a large bowl, followed by a pinch of salt. Continue layering in this fashion until all the cabbage and salt have been used.

3. Cover the cabbage bowl with a clean dish towel and allow it to rest on the countertop for 1 hour.

4. Using your hands, work the spice paste into the rested cabbage.

5. Stir in the green onion and radishes until they are evenly distributed.

6. Press the mixture into 3 half-quart jars, packing it as tightly as possible while leaving about an inch of headroom in each jar. You can use a muddle or fork to pack the jars.

7. Pour the liquid from the mixing bowl evenly into each jar, making sure the liquid covers the solid part of the kimchi but leaves about an inch of headroom.

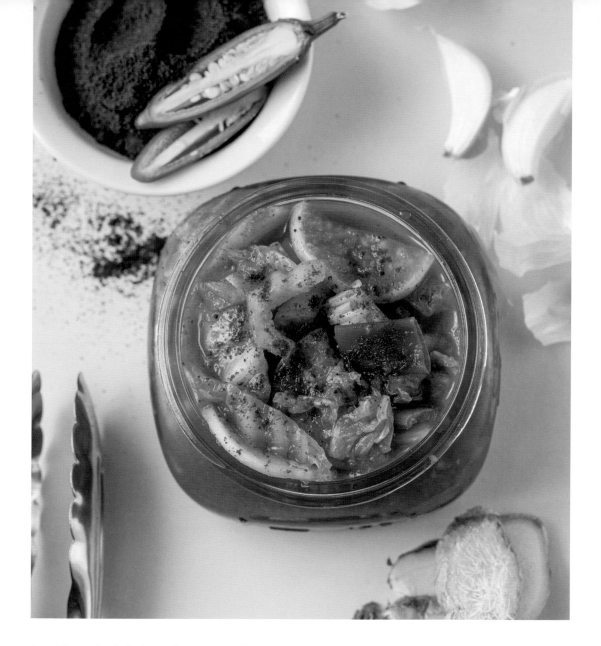

8. Place the lids loosely onto each jar and set the jars on a plate to catch any overflow.

9. Using a fork, pack the kimchi tightly into the bottom of the jars once or twice a day for the following 2 days.

10. You will notice air pockets and bubbles forming on day 2. This is normal and part of the fermentation process.

11. After 2 days of fermentation, the kimchi is ready to eat. Screw the lids on tight and keep in the fridge for up to a month.

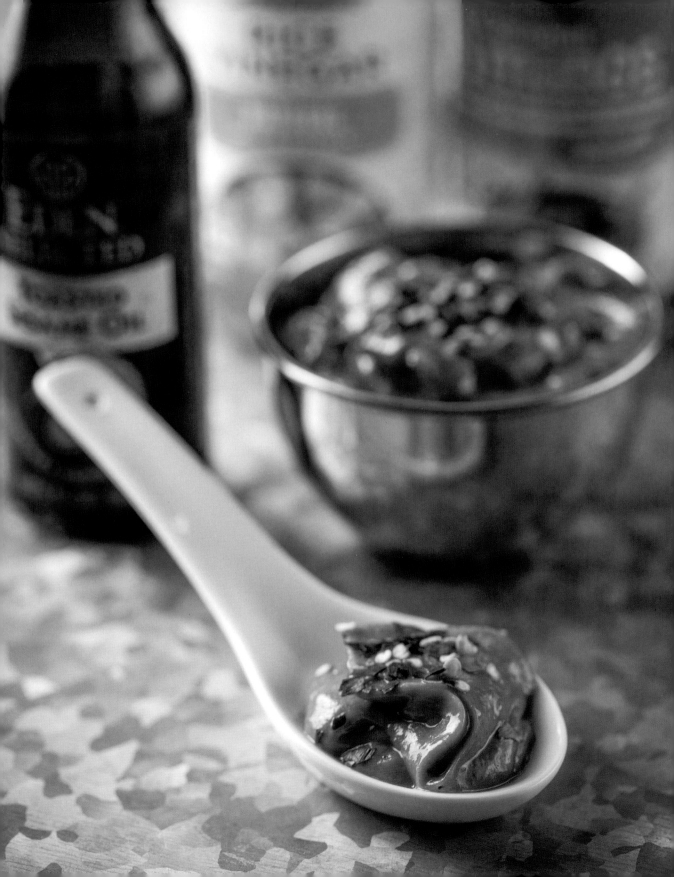

SPICY NUT BUTTER SAUCE

This Asian-inspired sauce is a family favorite. Keep it thick to use as a spread on sandwiches or wraps or thin it out to use as a salad dressing, over noodles, or as a sauce for your veggies. You will love it!

Yield: About 1 cup | *Serves 4 to 6*

½ cup almond, cashew, or peanut butter

3 tablespoons coconut aminos

2 tablespoons rice vinegar

1 tablespoon maple syrup

1 teaspoon toasted sesame oil

½ teaspoon crushed red pepper

1 large garlic clove, minced

½ teaspoon grated fresh ginger

Whisk all the ingredients to a smooth consistency in a medium-sized bowl. To thin the sauce, whisk in 1 tablespoon of water at a time until a pourable consistency is achieved.

A seven-year study found that stage III colon cancer survivors who ate at least two ounces of tree nuts per week (about seven almonds or walnuts per day) were 42 percent less likely to have their cancer return and 57 percent less likely to die from cancer than those who did not eat nuts. The benefit applied only to those eating tree nuts (almonds, walnuts, Brazil nuts, pistachios, and cashews) but not peanuts.[74]

SUPER SOFRITO

Puerto Rican sofrito, also known as *recaito*, is a condiment made with anticancer superstars garlic and onions combined with tomatoes, peppers, and various herbs and spices. Our Super Sofrito is super potent and super simple to make. Add sofrito to soups, stews, pasta, and rice bowls.

Yield: 1 to 1¼ cups

2 Roma or other medium tomatoes

1 cup loosely packed cilantro

1 red or yellow bell pepper, cored and seeded

2 green bell peppers, cored and seeded

1 tablespoon apple cider vinegar

2 medium red onions

1 bulb (10 to 12 cloves) garlic, peeled

Juice of ¼ lemon

½ teaspoon sea salt

1 teaspoon paprika (optional)

Blend all the ingredients in the work bowl of a food processor into a smooth paste similar to the consistency of pesto. Can be stored in the refrigerator for up to 3 days.

A study on Puerto Rican women found that those who consumed sofrito once or more per day had a 67 percent decreased risk of breast cancer compared to those who never consumed sofrito.[75]

A study in China found that adults who ate the highest amount of allium vegetables (garlic, onions, and leeks) had up to a 79 percent reduced risk of developing colorectal cancer compared to those who consumed the lowest amounts.[76]

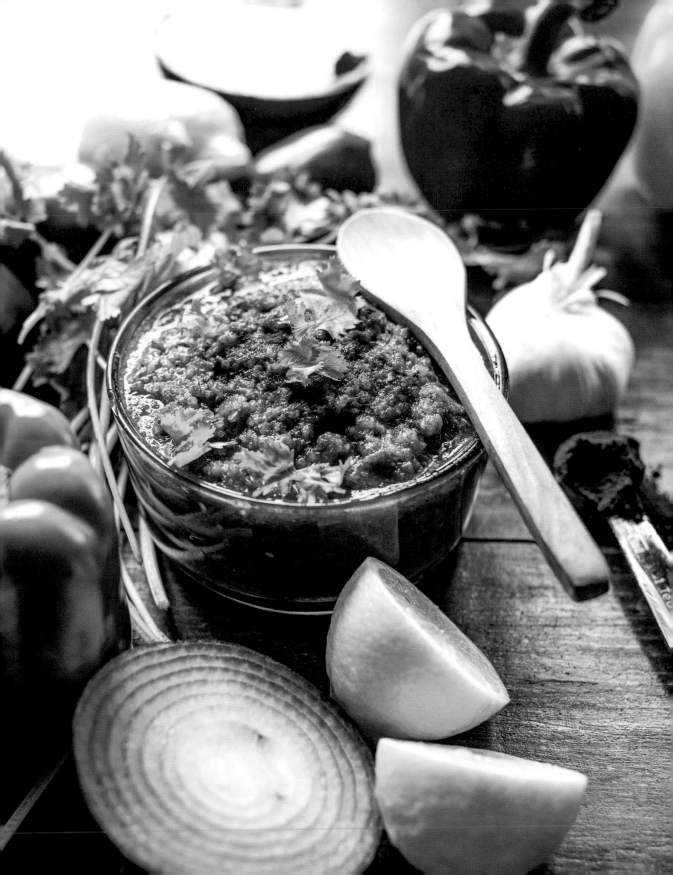

PEACH BBQ SAUCE

This sauce fuses two classic flavors of the American South with some of our favorite anticancer spices. This is a super-delish addition to your favorite veggies and bowls.

Yield: 1 quart

1 tablespoon toasted sesame oil

1 medium white onion, diced (about 1 ½ cups)

2 tablespoons sweet paprika

1 teaspoon granulated garlic

1 teaspoon black pepper

1 teaspoon dried thyme

½ teaspoon powdered ginger

3 medium peaches, pitted but not peeled (about 1 ½ cups)

One 15-ounce can tomato sauce

½ cup apple cider vinegar

1 tablespoon maple syrup

2 tablespoons grainy mustard

1 medium jalapeño, minced (optional)

1. Place the oil and onion in a medium saucepan over medium-high heat and sauté for 5 minutes, or until the onion is translucent and begins to brown.

2. Combine the paprika, garlic, pepper, thyme, ginger, peaches, tomato sauce, vinegar, maple syrup, mustard, and jalapeño, if using, in a blender until smooth.

3. Transfer the blended peach mixture to the saucepan, allow the mixture to heat through, then reduce the heat and simmer for 20 minutes.

4. Use immediately. The sauce can be stored in the fridge for up to 1 week, or in the freezer for up to 6 months.

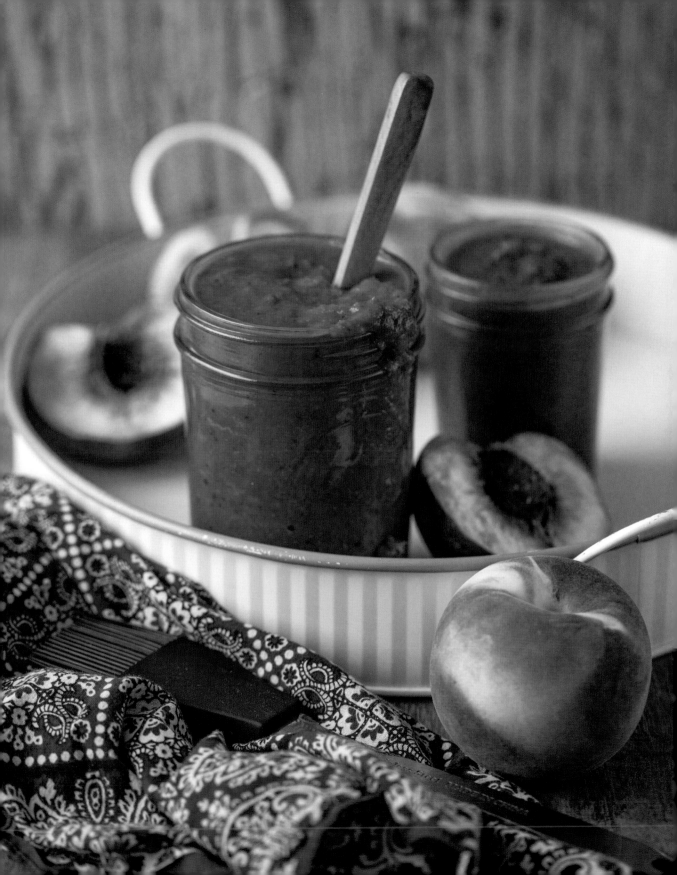

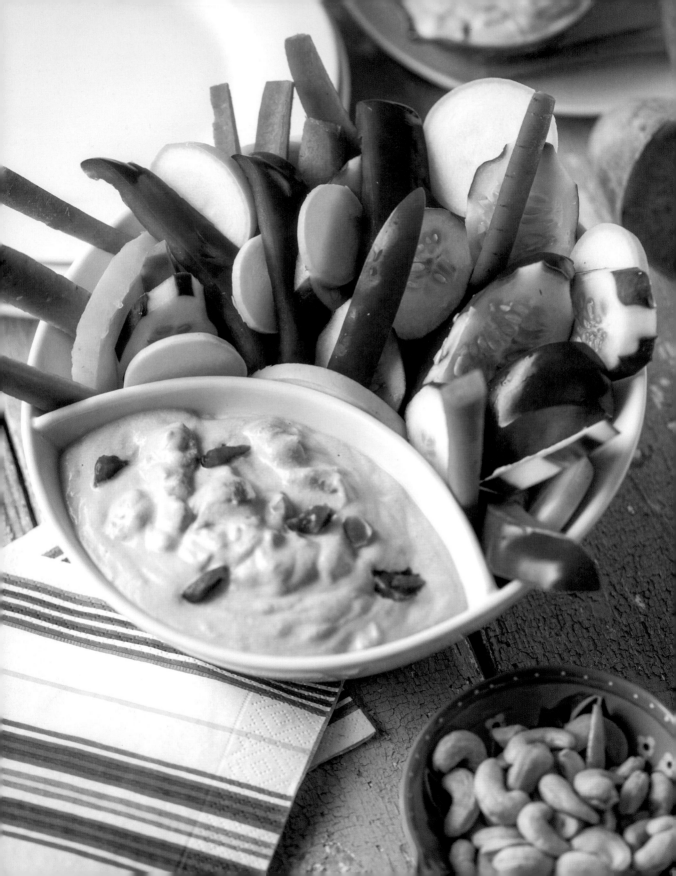

NACHO CHEEZE DIP

Our cheesy cheese-free dip made with sweet potatoes, cashews, and nutritional yeast is unbelievably yummy. It's great as a party dip, and no one will know it's made from plants!

Yield: About 2 cups | *Serves 6*

½ cup peeled, diced, and cooked sweet potato (from about ½ a medium sweet potato)

1 cup raw cashews

½ cup water, plus more if needed

2 garlic cloves

1 teaspoon cumin

½ teaspoon ground coriander

½ teaspoon sea salt

Juice of 1 medium lime

¼ cup nutritional yeast

1 large Roma tomato, diced (about 1 cup)

1 medium jalapeño, seeded and minced

Raw vegetables, for dipping

1. Bring a small pot filled halfway with water to a boil over high heat, add the sweet potato, and cook for 5 minutes, or until tender. Drain and set aside.

2. Blend the sweet potato and cashews in a blender. Add 1 tablespoon of water at a time if needed to get the mixture moving.

3. Let the mixture sit for 10 minutes to allow the cashews to soften.

4. Add the garlic, cumin, coriander, salt, lime juice, and nutritional yeast and blend until very smooth.

5. Pour the dip into a serving bowl and fold in the tomato and jalapeño pepper. Serve alongside, on top of, or stuffed into your favorite southwestern and Mexican-inspired dishes, including our Nacho-Style Sweet Potatoes (page 148).

SUPER SRIRACHA

This spicy, garlicky, and savory condiment goes with almost everything. Add a punch of flavor to your avocado toast, stew, tofu, or tacos. It really knows no boundaries.

Yield: 2 cups

1 quart red jalapeño peppers

¼ cup garlic cloves, peeled

⅛ cup apple cider vinegar

⅛ cup water

1 teaspoon sea salt

1. Combine all the ingredients in a blender until smooth.

2. Stir the mixture in a small saucepan over medium heat until heated through, about 10 minutes. This will mellow the garlic and sweeten the sauce.

3. Transfer to an airtight container and place in the fridge until ready to use.

NOTE: Our Super Sriracha will keep in the fridge for a month or in the freezer for six months.

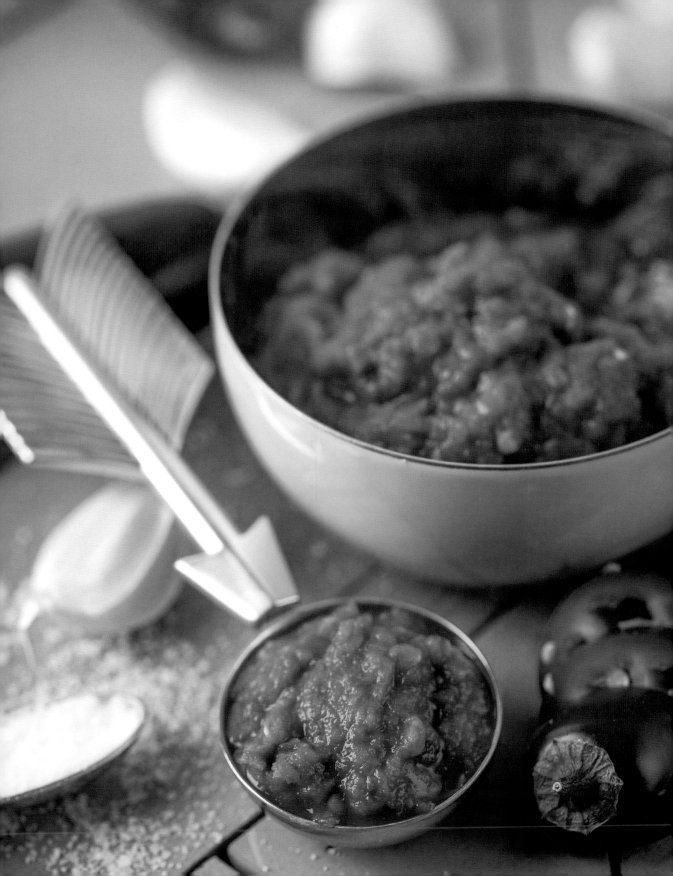

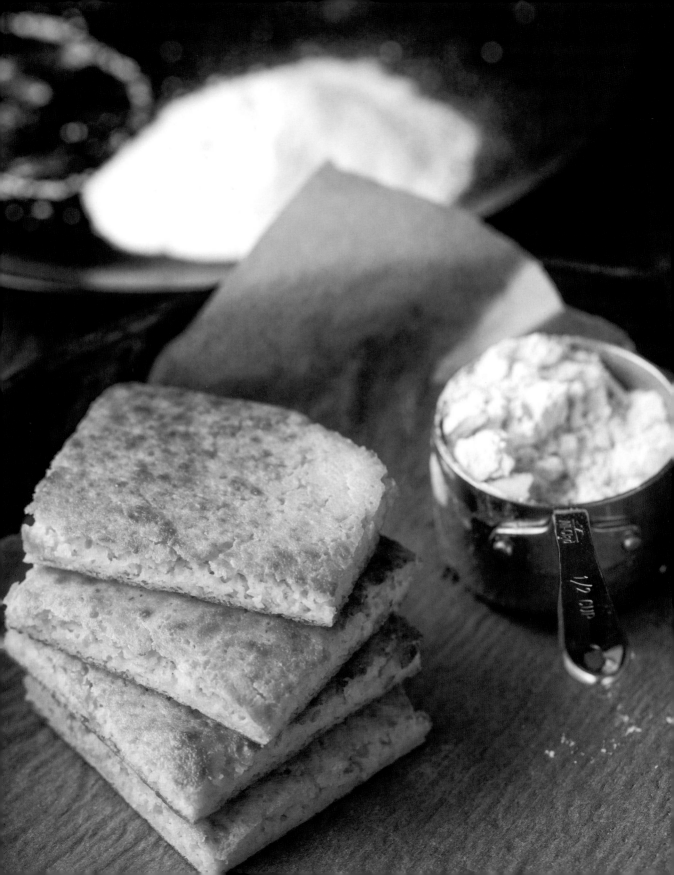

BEAN AND RICE FLATBREAD

This versatile flatbread made from garbanzo beans and rice is a delicious gluten-free bread, similar in texture and taste to cornbread. It's a perfect companion to soup or our Southern Veggie Plate (page 122) and also makes a fabulous pizza crust (page 152).

Yield: 1 flatbread | *Serves 4*

½ cup rice flour

1 cup garbanzo bean flour

1 teaspoon sea salt

2 ¼ teaspoons (1 packet) rapid-rise yeast

1 ¼ cups water

2 teaspoons extra-virgin olive oil

Leaves from 1 to 2 fresh sprigs of rosemary, to garnish (optional)

1. Preheat your oven to 425°F.

2. Whisk the rice flour, garbanzo bean flour, salt, yeast, and water in a large mixing bowl until there are no lumps, about the same consistency as pancake batter.

3. Coat a parchment-lined 12-inch skillet with olive oil.

4. Add the batter to the skillet, cover with a plate, and allow the batter to rise for 40 minutes.

5. Sprinkle the fresh rosemary sprigs on top, if desired.

6. Bake for 20 to 25 minutes or until the top of the bread is lightly browned.

JUICER BROTH

Here's a quick way to make a fresh, flavorful vegetable broth with your juicer.

Yield: 6 cups

1 celery stalk

1 bunch parsley

1 pound carrots

1 medium white or sweet onion, peeled

5 medium Roma tomatoes

1 medium bell pepper, seeded

1 teaspoon apple cider vinegar

¼ teaspoon sea salt

1. Feed the celery, parsley, carrots, onion, tomatoes, and bell pepper into your juicer. Add the apple cider vinegar and salt to the juice mixture.

2. Store in the fridge if you plan on using it within 5 days or store in the freezer for up to 6 months.

PRO TIP: This is a rich, flavorful juice/broth. Diluting with 2 cups filtered water will increase the yield and produce a milder-flavored broth that is comparable to a store-bought vegetable broth.

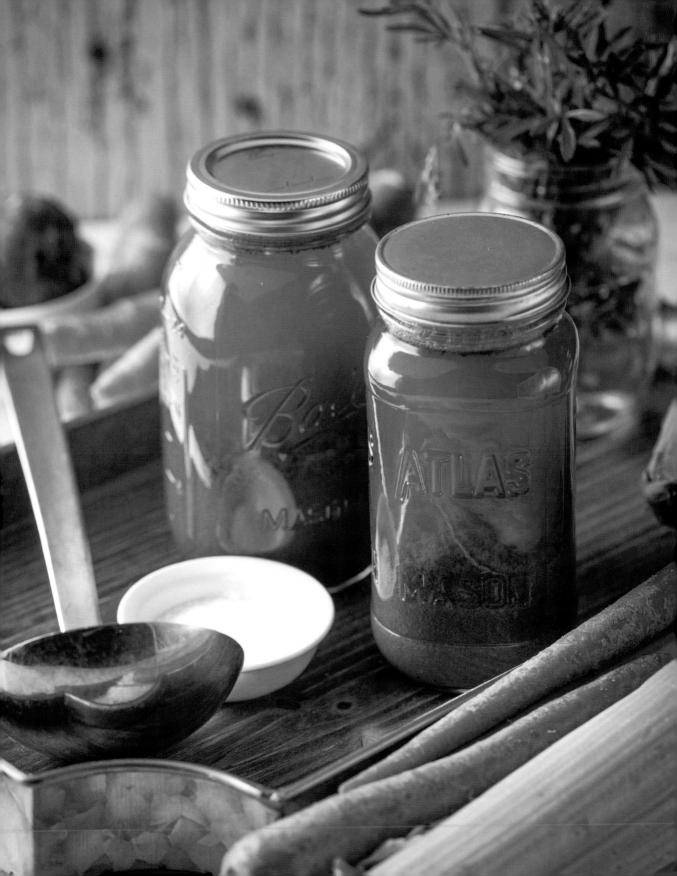

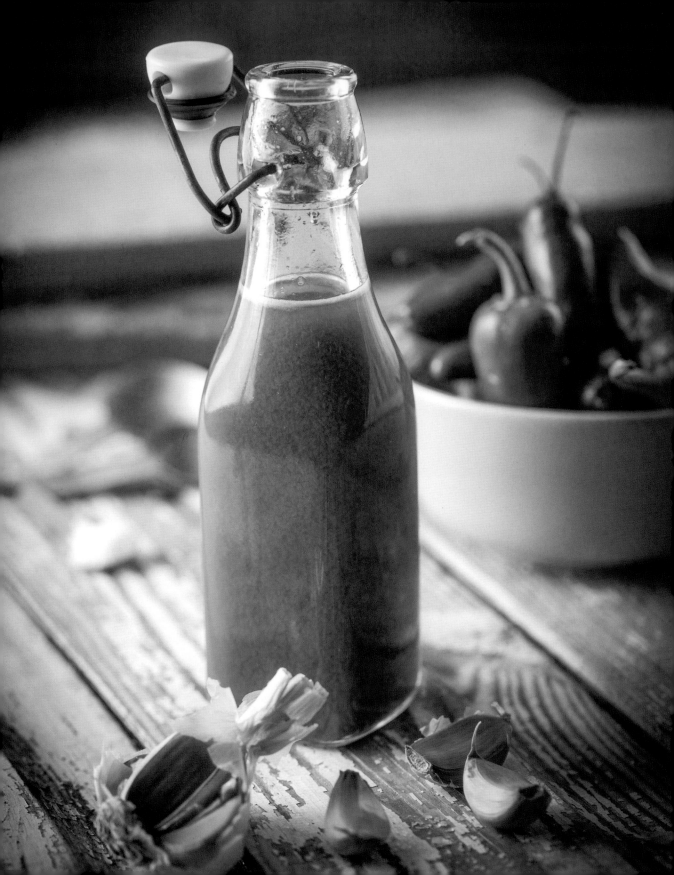

JUICER HOT SAUCE

Here's how to make a fresh and fiery hot sauce with your juicer. As you know, peppers vary in intensity. Make sure you check the heat before you drizzle on food.

Yield: About 1 cup

2 to 3 garlic cloves

2 cups fresh jalapeño peppers

½ cup apple cider vinegar

¼ teaspoon sea salt

¼ cup water

1. Run the garlic cloves and peppers through your juicer; they should yield about ½ cup juice.

2. Funnel the garlic-pepper juice, apple cider vinegar, salt, and water into a resealable container and shake until the salt dissolves.

3. The hot sauce can be stored in the fridge for up to a month.

NOTE: For a medium hot sauce, use 2 cups poblano peppers. For a milder hot sauce, use 2 cups green bell peppers and 1 medium jalapeño or serrano pepper.

PRO TIP: Make the hot sauce right after making the veggie broth so you don't have to clean your juicer twice.

Capsaicin is the active compound in hot peppers that makes them hot. Capsaicin has been shown to alter the expression of several genes involved in cancer cell survival, growth, angiogenesis, and metastasis. Like curcumin in turmeric, capsaicin has been found to target multiple signaling pathways, oncogenes, and tumor-suppressor genes in various types of cancer models.[77]

EASY BAKED TOFU

Organic tofu can be a great addition to rice, pasta, and veggie dishes. Works beautifully with the Veggie Stir-Up (page 118).

Yield: 1½ pounds | *Serves 6 to 8*

2 blocks extra-firm tofu, drained and cubed

1. Preheat your oven to 350°F.

2. Space out the tofu squares on a parchment-lined baking sheet so they do not touch.

3. Bake for 20 minutes (or up to 30 minutes for a firmer texture).

NOTE: Most soy grown in the U.S. is genetically modified and sprayed with glyphosate-based herbicide. To avoid this, buy organic tofu.

PRO TIP: Cooking tofu this way helps it absorb any sauces or spices you pair it with. Bake your tofu at the beginning of the week and have it at the ready for soups, salads, bowls, and stir-fries. You can jazz it up with our Spicy Nut Butter Sauce page 203 or Orange-Ginger Sauce page 119.

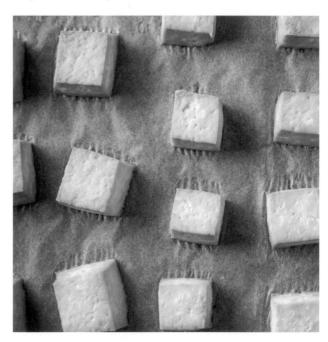

Soybeans are rich in anticancer flavones, and multiple studies have found that the consumption of soy reduces a woman's risk of breast cancer[78] and a man's risk of prostate cancer.[79] A study on breast cancer patients found that women who consumed the most soy (up to 11 grams per day) had a 34 percent decreased risk of recurrence and a 33 percent reduced risk of death compared to those who consumed the least.[80] For reference, 11 grams of soy per day is roughly one cup of soybeans, 6 ounces of tofu, or 8 to 12 ounces of soy milk.

MAPLE SUSHI RICE

This is our version of traditional Japanese sushi rice. Enjoy with veggies or in our DIY Sushi Tacos (page 144).

Yield: 5 cups | *Serves 4 to 6*

---

2 cups brown or white sushi rice, rinsed in a strainer

2 cups water

1 tablespoon rice vinegar

1 tablespoon maple syrup

1 teaspoon sea salt

1. Add the sushi rice and water to your rice cooker and choose the "white rice" setting. Alternately, follow the cooking instructions on the package.

2. Whisk the vinegar, maple syrup, and salt in a small bowl.

3. Fold the vinegar mixture into the cooked rice.

4. Transfer to a bowl and cover with a towel if you plan to use the rice immediately or refrigerate up to 5 days.

SHAKE & BAKE CHICKPEAS

These toasted chickpeas, spiced with our Anticancer Sprinkle, put the nutritional smackdown on traditional croutons. Once you try them, you'll be a fan for life.

Yield: 1 cup | *Serves 4*

One 15-ounce can chickpeas, drained, or 1½ cups cooked chickpeas

1 tablespoon Anticancer Sprinkle (page 19)

2 teaspoons extra-virgin olive oil

1. Preheat your oven to 400°F.

2. Place the chickpeas and the Anticancer Sprinkle in a closed container and shake until the chickpeas are evenly coated.

3. Spread the chickpeas in a single layer on a parchment-lined baking sheet and drizzle with olive oil.

4. Bake 20 minutes for a softer chewy consistency or 40 to 45 minutes for more crunch, shaking the baking sheet halfway through to ensure even cooking.

5. Allow the chickpeas to cool completely.

6. Enjoy as a snack or as a spicy topping for your favorite salads, soups, and main dishes.

PRO TIP: Double the recipe and store in a sealed container, unrefrigerated, for up to a week. They are always gone before they have a chance to go bad. Our kids love these as a lunch-box snack.

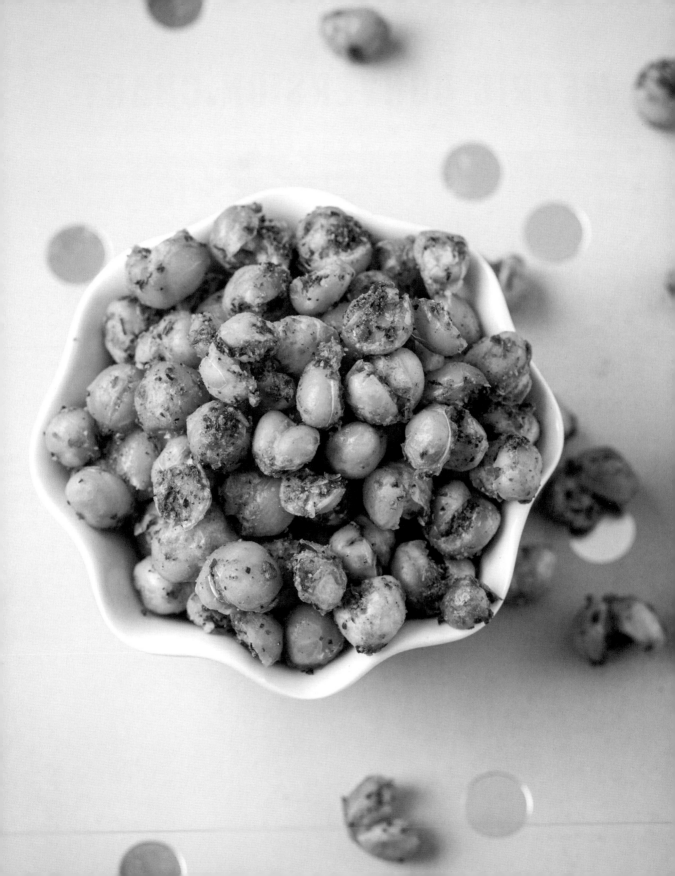

METRIC CONVERSION CHART

Standard Cup	Fine Powder (e.g., flour)	Grain (e.g., rice)	Granular (e.g., sugar)	Liquid Solids (e.g., butter)	Liquid (e.g., milk)
1	140 g	150 g	190 g	200 g	240 ml
³/₄	105 g	113 g	143 g	150 g	180 ml
²/₃	93 g	100 g	125 g	133 g	160 ml
¹/₂	70 g	75 g	95 g	100 g	120 ml
¹/₃	47 g	50 g	63 g	67 g	80 ml
¹/₄	35 g	38 g	48 g	50 g	60 ml
¹/₈	18 g	19 g	24 g	25 g	30 ml

Useful Equivalents for Cooking/Oven Temperatures

Process	Fahrenheit	Celsius	Gas Mark
Freeze Water	32° F	0° C	
Room Temperature	68° F	20° C	
Boil Water	212° F	100° C	
Bake	325° F	160° C	3
	350° F	180° C	4
	375° F	190° C	5
	400° F	200° C	6
	425° F	220° C	7
	450° F	230° C	8
Broil			Grill

Useful Equivalents for Liquid Ingredients by Volume

¹/₄ tsp			1 ml
¹/₂ tsp			2 ml
1 tsp			5 ml
3 tsp	1 tbsp	¹/₂ fl oz	15 ml
	2 tbsp	¹/₈ cup	1 fl oz	30 ml
	4 tbsp	¹/₄ cup	2 fl oz	60 ml
	5¹/₃ tbsp	¹/₃ cup	3 fl oz	80 ml
	8 tbsp	¹/₂ cup	4 fl oz	120 ml
	10²/₃ tbsp	²/₃ cup	5 fl oz	160 ml
	12 tbsp	³/₄ cup	6 fl oz	180 ml
	16 tbsp	1 cup	8 fl oz	240 ml
	1 pt	2 cups	16 fl oz	480 ml
	1 qt	4 cups	32 fl oz	960 ml
			33 fl oz	1000 ml	1 L

Useful Equivalents for Dry Ingredients by Weight

(To convert ounces to grams, multiply the number of ounces by 30.)

1 oz	¹/₁₆ lb	30 g
4 oz	¹/₄ lb	120 g
8 oz	¹/₂ lb	240 g
12 oz	³/₄ lb	360 g
16 oz	1 lb	480 g

Useful Equivalents for Length

(To convert inches to centimeters, multiply the number of inches by 2.5.)

1 in			2.5 cm	
6 in	¹/₂ ft		15 cm	
12 in	1 ft		30 cm	
36 in	3 ft	1 yd	90 cm	
40 in			100 cm	1 m

ENDNOTES

Introduction

1. Tetsushi Yamamoto, et al., "Inhibitory Effect of Maple Syrup on the Cell Growth and Invasion of Human Colorectal Cancer Cells," *Oncology Reports* 33, no. 4 (April 2015): 1579–1584. https://www.ncbi .nlm.nih.gov/pmc/articles/PMC4358083/#!po=55.7143.

2. Katherine M. Phillips, et al., "Total Antioxidant Content of Alternatives to Refined Sugar," *Journal of the American Dietetic Association* 109, no. 1 (January 2009): 64–71. https://pubmed.ncbi.nlm.nih.gov/ 19103324/.

3. Peter Grandics, "Cancer: A Single Disease with a Multitude of Manifestations?" *Journal of Carcinogenesis* 2, no. 9 (2003). https://www.ncbi.nlm.nih.gov/pmc/articles/PMC305362/#__sec3title.

4. Ibid.

5. Liza Oates, et al., "Reduction in Urinary Organophosphate Pesticide Metabolites in Adults After a Week-Long Organic Diet," *Journal of Environmental Research* 132 (June 2014): 105–11. https://www.ncbi.nlm .nih.gov/pubmed/24769399 (accessed April 2018).

6. Zhi-Yong Yang, et al., "Effects of Home Preparation on Pesticide Residues in Cabbage," *Food Control* 18, no. 12 (December 2007): 1484–1487. https://www.sciencedirect .com/science/article/pii/ S0956713506002696 (accessed May 2018).

7. Simona Bo, et al., "Is the Timing of Caloric Intake Associated with Variation in Diet-Induced Thermogenesis and in the Metabolic Pattern? A Randomized Cross-Over Study," *International Journal of Obesity and Related Metabolic Disorders* 39, no. 12 (December 2015): 1689–95. https://pubmed.ncbi.nlm .nih.gov/26219416/.

8. Catherine R. Marinac, et al., "Prolonged Nightly Fasting and Breast Cancer Prognosis," *JAMA Oncology* 2, no. 8 (August 1, 2016): 1049–1055. https://pubmed.ncbi.nlm.nih.gov/27032109/.

9. International Agency for Research on Cancer, World Health Organization, "IARC Monographs Evaluate Consumption of Red Meat and Processed Meat," press release no. 240 (October 26, 2015). https://www .iarc.who.int/wp-content/uploads/2018/07/pr240_E.pdf.

10. International Agency for Research on Cancer, World Health Organization, "Q&A on the Carcinogenicity of the Consumption of Red Meat and Processed Meat," (2015). https://www.iarc.who .int/wp-content/uploads/2018/11/Monographs-QA_Vol114.pdf.

11. Véronique Bouvard, et al., "Carcinogenicity of Consumption of Red and Processed Meat," *Lancet Oncology* 16, no. 16 (December 2015): 1599–600. https://pubmed.ncbi.nlm.nih.gov/26514947/.

12. Giuseppe Lippi, et al., "Meat Consumption and Cancer Risk: A Critical Review of Published Meta-Analysis," *Critical Reviews in Oncology/Hematology* 97 (January 2016): 1–14. https://www.sciencedirect .com/science/article/abs/pii/S1040842815300780.

13. Morgan E. Levine, et al., "Low Protein Intake Is Associated with a Major Reduction in IGF-1, Cancer, and Overall Mortality in the 65 and Younger but Not Older Population," *Cell Metabolism* 19, no. 3 (March 4, 2014): 407–17. https://pubmed.ncbi.nlm.nih.gov/24606898/.

14. Jae Jeong Yang, et al., "Dietary Fat Intake and Lung Cancer Risk: A Pooled Analysis," *Journal of Clinical Oncology* 35, no. 26 (September 10, 2017): 3055–3064. https://pubmed.ncbi.nlm.nih.gov/28742456/.

15. Semir Beyaz, et al., "High-Fat Diet Enhances Stemness and Tumorigenicity of Intestinal Progenitors," *Nature* 531 (March 2, 2016): 53–58. https://www.nature.com/articles/nature17173.

16. Emma H. Allot, et al., "Saturated Fat Intake and Prostate Cancer Aggressiveness: Results from the Population-Based North Carolina-Louisiana Prostate Cancer Project," *Prostate Cancer and Prostatic Diseases* 20, no. 1 (March 2017): 48–54. https://pubmed.ncbi.nlm.nih.gov/27595916/.

17. Hui Xia, et al., "Meta-Analysis of Saturated Fatty Acid Intake and Breast Cancer Risk," *Medicine* 94, no. 52 (December 2015): e2391. https://www.ncbi.nlm.nih.gov/pmc/articles/PMC5291630/.

18. Sarah F. Brennan, et al., "Dietary Fat and Breast Cancer Mortality: A Systematic Review and Meta-Analysis," *Critical Reviews in Food Science Nutrition* 57, no. 10 (July 3, 2017): 1999–2008. https://pubmed.ncbi.nlm.nih.gov/25692500/.

19. Jia Hu, et al., "Dietary Cholesterol Intake and Cancer," *Annals of Oncology* 23, no. 2 (February 2012): 491–500. https://pubmed.ncbi.nlm.nih.gov/21543628/.

20. Binlu Huang, et al., "Cholesterol Metabolism in Cancer: Mechanisms and Therapeutic Opportunities," *Nature Metabolism* 2 (February 10, 2020): 132–141. https://www.nature.com/articles/s42255-020-0174-0.

21. Rudolf Kaaks, "Nutrition, Insulin, IGF-1 Metabolism and Cancer Risk: A Summary of Epidemiological Evidence," Novartis Foundation Symposium 262 (2004): 247–60; discussion 260–68. https://pubmed.ncbi.nlm.nih.gov/15562834/.

22. R. James Barnard, et al., "Effects of a Low-Fat, High-Fiber Diet and Exercise Program on Breast Cancer Risk Factors in Vivo and Tumor Cell Growth and Apoptosis in Vitro," *Nutrition and Cancer* 55, no. 1 (2006): 28–34. https://pubmed.ncbi.nlm.nih.gov/16965238/.

23. Barbara C. Halpern, et al., "The Effect of Replacement of Methionine by Homocystine on Survival of Malignant and Normal Adult Mammalian Cells in Culture," *Proceedings of the National Academy of Sciences of the United States of America* 71, no. 4 (April 1974): 1133–1136. https://www.ncbi.nlm.nih.gov/pmc/articles/PMC388177/.

24. Paul Cavuoto and Michael F. Fenech, "A Review of Methionine Dependency and the Role of Methionine Restriction in Cancer Growth Control and Life-Span Extension," *Cancer Treatment Reviews* 38, no. 6 (October 2012): 726–36. https://pubmed.ncbi.nlm.nih.gov/22342103/.

25. Mary H. Ward, et al., "Heme Iron from Meat and Risk of Adenocarcinoma of the Esophagus and Stomach," *European Journal of Cancer Prevention* 21, no. 2 (March 2012): 134–8. https://pubmed.ncbi.nlm.nih.gov/22044848/.

26. Nadia M. Bastide, et al., "Heme Iron from Meat and Risk of Colorectal Cancer: A Meta-Analysis and a Review of the Mechanisms Involved," *Cancer Prevention Research* 4, no. 2 (February 2011): 177–84. https://pubmed.ncbi.nlm.nih.gov/21209396/.

27. Vicky C. Chang, et al., "Iron Intake, Body Iron Status, and Risk of Breast Cancer: A Systematic Review and Meta-Analysis," *BMC Cancer* 19, no. 543 (2019). https://bmccancer.biomedcentral.com/articles/10.1186/s12885-019-5642-0.

28. Suna Ji, et al., "Developmental Changes in the Level of Free and Conjugated Sialic Acids, Neu5Ac, Neu5Gc and KDN in Different Organs of Pig: A LC-MS/MS Quantitative Analyses. *Glycoconjugate Journal* 34 (2016): 21–30. https://link.springer.com/article/10.1007/s10719-016-9724-9.

29. University of California - Davis Health System, "Neu5Gc in Red Meat and Organs May Pose a Significant Health Hazard," ScienceDaily (October 19, 2016). https://www.sciencedaily.com/releases/2016/10/161019160201.htm.

30. Carrie R. Daniel, et al., "Large Prospective Investigation of Meat Intake, Related Mutagens, and Risk of Renal Cell Carcinoma," *American Journal of Clinical Nutrition* 95, no. 1 (January 2012): 155–62. https://pubmed.ncbi.nlm.nih.gov/22170360/.

31. Jun Wang, et al., "Carcinogen Metabolism Genes, Red Meat and Poultry Intake, and Colorectal Cancer Risk," *International Journal of Cancer* 130, no. 8 (April 15, 2012): 1898–907. https://pubmed.ncbi.nlm.nih.gov/21618522/.

32. Eduardo De Stefani, et al., "Meat Consumption, Meat Cooking and Risk of Lung Cancer among Uruguayan Men," *Asian Pacific Journal of Cancer Prevention* 11, no. 6 (2010): 1713–7. https://pubmed.ncbi.nlm.nih.gov/21338220/.

33. Esther M. John, et al., "Meat Consumption, Cooking Practices, Meat Mutagens and Risk of Prostate Cancer," *Nutrition and Cancer* 63, no. 4 (2011): 525–537. https://www.ncbi.nlm.nih.gov/pmc/articles/PMC3516139/.

34. Kristin E. Anderson, et al., "Pancreatic Cancer Risk: Associations with Meat-Derived Carcinogen Intake in the Prostate, Lung, Colorectal, and Ovarian Cancer Screening Trial (PLCO) Cohort," *Molecular Carcinogens* 51, no. 1 (January 2012): 128–137. https://www.ncbi.nlm.nih.gov/pmc/articles/PMC3516181/.

35. Donghui Li, et al., "Dietary Mutagen Exposure and Risk of Pancreatic Cancer," *Cancer Epidemiology, Biomarkers & Prevention* 6, no. 4 (April 2007): 655–661. https://www.ncbi.nlm.nih.gov/pmc/articles/PMC1892159/.

36. Stephen J. D. O'Keefe, et al., "Rarity of Colon Cancer in Africans Is Associated with Low Animal Product Consumption, Not Fiber," *American Journal of Gastroenterology* 94, no. 5 (May 1999): 1373–80. https://pubmed.ncbi.nlm.nih.gov/10235221/.

37. Ivana Vucenik and AbulKalam M. Shamsuddin, "Protection against Cancer by Dietary IP6 and Inositol," *Nutrition and Cancer* 55, no. 2 (2006): 109–25. https://pubmed.ncbi.nlm.nih.gov/17044765/.

38. Irene Darmadi-Blackberry, et al., "Legumes: The Most Important Dietary Predictor of Survival in Older People of Different Ethnicities," *Asia Pacific Journal of Clinical Nutrition* 13, no. 2 (2004): 217–20. https://pubmed.ncbi.nlm.nih.gov/15228991/.

39. Yu-Mei Hsueh, et al., "Serum Beta-Carotene Level, Arsenic Methylation Capability, and Incidence of Skin Cancer," *Cancer Epidemiology, Biomarkers & Prevention* 6, no. 8 (August 1997): 589–96. https://pubmed.ncbi.nlm.nih.gov/9264271/.

40. Michael Greger, "Benefits of Turmeric for Arsenic Exposure," NutritionFacts.org 38 (September 20, 2017): https://nutritionfacts.org/video/benefits-of-turmeric-for-arsenic-exposure/.

41. Xiao-Qin Wang, et al., "Review of Salt Consumption and Stomach Cancer Risk: Epidemiological and Biological Evidence," *World Journal of Gastroenterology* 15, no. 18 (May 14, 2009): 2204–2213. https://www.ncbi.nlm.nih.gov/pmc/articles/PMC2682234/.

42. Joe M. McCord, "Analysis of Superoxide Dismutase Activity," *Current Protocols in Toxicology* 7, no. 1 (May 2001): 7.3. https://pubmed.ncbi.nlm.nih.gov/23045062/.

43. Katarzyna Jobin, et al., "A High-Salt Diet Compromises Antibacterial Neutrophil Responses through Hormonal Perturbation," *Science Translational Medicine* 12, no. 536 (March 25, 2020): eaay3850. https://stm.sciencemag.org/content/12/536/eaay3850.

44. Weiwei Lin, et al., "Meta-Analysis of the Effects of Indoor Nitrogen Dioxide and Gas Cooking on Asthma and Wheeze in Children," *International Journal of Epidemiology* 42, no. 6 (December 2013): 1724–1737. https://academic.oup.com/ije/article/42/6/1724/737113.

45. Donghai Liang, et al., "Urban Air Pollution May Enhance COVID-19 Case-Fatality and Mortality Rates in the United States," *The Innovation* 1, no. 3 (November 25, 2020): 100047. https://www.cell.com/the-innovation/fulltext/S2666-6758(20)30050-3#%20.

Part I

46. Yi-Fang Chu, et al., "Antioxidant and Antiproliferative Activities of Common Vegetables," *Journal of Agriculture and Food Chemistry* 50, no. 23 (October 10, 2002): 6910–6916. https://doi.org/10.1021/jf020665f.

47. Mohammed El Haouari, et al., "Anticancer Molecular Mechanisms of Oleocanthal," *Phytotherapy Research* 34, no 11 (November 2020): 2820–2834. https://pubmed.ncbi.nlm.nih.gov/32449241/.

48. Liping Guo, et al., "Effect of Freezing Methods on Sulforaphane Formation in Broccoli Sprouts," *RSC Advances* 41, no. 5 (2015): 32290–32297. https://pubs.rsc.org/en/content/articlelanding/2015/ra/c5ra03403e#!divAbstract.

Fresh Juices

49. Edward Giovannucci, "Tomatoes, Tomato-Based Products, Lycopene, and Cancer: Review of the Epidemiologic Literature," *Journal of the National Cancer Institute* 91, no. 4 (February 17, 1999): 317–331. https://academic.oup.com/jnci/article/91/4/31⁷/2543924.

50. Harvard T.H. Chan School of Public Health, "Eating More Whole Grains Linked with Lower Mortality Rates," press release (June 13, 2016). https://www.hsph.harvard.edu/news/press-releases/whole-grains-lower-mortality-rates/.

Smoothies

51. Lisa S. McAnulty, et al., "Six Weeks Daily Ingestion of Whole Blueberry Powder Increases Natural Killer Cell Counts and Reduces Arterial Stiffness in Sedentary Males and Females," *Nutritional Research* 34, no. 7 (July 2014): 577–84. https://pubmed.ncbi.nlm.nih.gov/25150116/.

Part II

Rise and Shine

52. Yaser Sharif, et al., "Legume and Nuts Consumption in Relation to Odds of Breast Cancer: A Case-Control Study," *Nutrition and Cancer* 73, no. 5 (2021): 750–759. https://pubmed.ncbi.nlm.nih.gov/32475175/.

53. Peng-Gao Li, et al., "Anticancer Effects of Sweet Potato Protein on Human Colorectal Cancer Cells," *World Journal of Gastroenterology* 19, no. 21 (June 7, 2013): 3300–8. https://pubmed.ncbi.nlm.nih.gov/23745032/.

Salads

54. Saravana Kumar Jaganathan, et al., "Chemopreventive Effect of Apple and Berry Fruits against Colon Cancer," *World Journal of Gastroenterology* 20, no. 45 (December 7, 2014): 17029–17036. https://www.ncbi.nlm.nih.gov/pmc/articles/PMC4258571/.

55. Yaser Sharif, et al., "Legume and Nuts Consumption in Relation to Odds of Breast Cancer: A Case-Control Study," *Nutrition and Cancer* 73, no. 5 (2021): 750–759. https://pubmed.ncbi.nlm.nih.gov/32475175/.

Soups and Sides

56. Min Zhang, et al., "Dietary Intakes of Mushrooms and Green Tea Combine to Reduce the Risk of Breast Cancer in Chinese Women," *International Journal of Cancer* 124, no. 6 (March 15, 2009): 1404–8. https://www.ncbi.nlm.nih.gov/pubmed/19048616 (accessed April 2018).

57. Birgit Wassermann, et al., "An Apple a Day: Which Bacteria Do We Eat with Organic and Conventional Apples?" *Frontiers in Microbiology* 10 (2019): 1629. https://www.frontiersin.org/articles/10.3389/fmicb.2019.01629/full.

58. Kuzhuvelil B. Harikumar, et al., "Sesamin Manifests Chemopreventive Effects through the Suppression of NF-Kappa B-Regulated Cell Survival, Proliferation, Invasion, and Angiogenic Gene Products," *Molecular Cancer Research* 8, no. 5 (May 2010): 751–61. https://pubmed.ncbi.nlm.nih.gov/20460401/.

59. Rachel S. Rosenberg, et al., "Modulation of Androgen and Progesterone Receptors by Phytochemicals in Breast Cancer Cell Lines," *Biochemical and Biophysical Research Communications* 248, no. 3 (August 1998): 935–39. https://pubmed.ncbi.nlm.nih.gov/9704030/ (accessed April 2018).

60. Xin Cai and Xuan Liu, "Inhibition of Thr-55 Phosphorylation Restores p53 Nuclear Localization and Sensitizes Cancer Cells to DNA Damage," *Proceedings of the National Academy of Sciences of the United States of America* 105, no. 44 (November 4, 2008): 16958–63. http://www.pnas.org/content/105/44/16958 (accessed April 2018).

Mains

61. Andrew Reynolds, et al., "Carbohydrate Quality and Human Health: A Series of Systematic Reviews and Meta-Analyses," *Lancet* 393, no. 10170 (February 2, 2019): 434–445. https://www.thelancet.com/journals/lancet/article/PIIS0140-6736(18)31809-9/fulltext.

62. Mei Dong, et al., "Phytochemicals of Black Bean Seed Coats: Isolation, Structure Elucidation, and Their Antiproliferative and Antioxidative Activities," *Journal of Agricultural and Food Chemistry* 55, no. 15 (July 25, 2007): 6044–51. https://pubmed.ncbi.nlm.nih.gov/17602653/.

63. Katya Chobotova, et al., "Bromelain's Activity and Potential as an Anti-Cancer Agent: Current Evidence and Perspectives," *Cancer Letters* 290, no. 2 (April 28, 2010): 148–56. https://pubmed.ncbi.nlm.nih.gov/19700238/.

64. Kosuke Nishi, et al, "Immunostimulatory in Vitro and in Vivo Effects of a Water-Soluble Extract from Kale," *Bioscience, Biotechnology, and Biochemistry* 75, no. 1 (2011): 40–6. https://pubmed.ncbi.nlm.nih.gov/21228486/.

65. Isabella Savini, et al., "Origanum vulgare Induces Apoptosis in Human Colon Cancer Caco2 Cells," *Nutrition and Cancer* 61, no. 3 (February 2009): 381–89. https://pubmed.ncbi.nlm.nih.gov/19373612/ (accessed Apr 2018).

66. Ladislav Vaśko, et al., "Comparison of Some Antioxidant Properties of Plant Extracts from Origanum vulgare, Salvia officinalis, Eleutherococcus senticosus and Stevia rebaudiana," *In Vitro Cellular & Developmental Biology—Animal* 50, no. 7 (August 2014): 614–22. https://www.ncbi.nlm.nih.gov/pubmed/24737278 (accessed Apr 2018).

67. Federation of American Societies for Experimental Biology (FASEB), "Component of Pizza Seasoning Herb Oregano Kills Prostate Cancer Cells," ScienceDaily (April 2012). www.sciencedaily.com/releases/2012/04/120424162224.htm (accessed Apr 2018).

68. Shiuan Chen et al, "Anti-Aromatase Activity of Phytochemicals in White Button Mushrooms (Agaricus bisporus)," *Cancer Research* 66.24 (Dec 2006): 12026–34. https://www.ncbi.nlm.nih.gov/pubmed/17178902 (accessed Apr 2018).

69. Sang Chul Jeong, et al., "Dietary Intake of *Agaricus bisporus* White Button Mushroom Accelerates Salivary Immunoglobulin A Secretion in Healthy Volunteers," *Nutrition* 28, no. 5 (May 2012): 527–31. http://www.nutritionjrnl.com/article/S0899-9007(11)00302-9/abstract (accessed April 2018).

Plant-Based Basics

70. Anne Berit, et al., "Effects of Orally Administered Yeast-Derived Beta-Glucans: A Review," *Molecular Nutrition & Food Research* 58, no. 1 (January 2014): 183–93. https://onlinelibrary.wiley.com/doi/full/10.1002/mnfr.201300338 (accessed April 2018).

71. Václav Větvička, et al., "Targeting of Natural Killer Cells to Mammary Carcinoma via Naturally Occurring Tumor Cell-Bound iC3b and Beta-Glucan-Primed CR3 (CD11b/CD18)," *Journal of Immunology* 159, no. 2 (July 15, 1997): 599–605. https://www.ncbi.nlm.nih.gov/pubmed/9218574 (accessed April 2018).

72. Gokhan Demir, et al., "Beta Glucan Induces Proliferation and Activation of Monocytes in Peripheral Blood of Patients with Advanced Breast Cancer," *International Immunopharmacology* 7, no. 1 (January 2007): 113–16. https://www.ncbi.nlm.nih.gov/pubmed/17161824 (accessed April 2018).

73. Monica H. Carlsen, et al., "The Total Antioxidant Content of More than 3100 Foods, Beverages, Spices, Herbs and Supplements Used Worldwide," *Nutrition Journal* 9, no. 3 (January 22, 2010). https://www.ncbi.nlm.nih.gov/pmc/articles/PMC2841576/.

74. Temidayo Fadelu, et al., "Nut Consumption and Survival in Stage III Colon Cancer Patients: Results from CALGB 89803 (Alliance)," *Journal of Clinical Oncology* 36, no. 11 (April 10, 2018): 1112–1120. https://pubmed.ncbi.nlm.nih.gov/29489429/.

75. Gauri Desai, et al., "Onion and Garlic Intake and Breast Cancer, a Case-Control Study in Puerto Rico," *Nutrition and Cancer* 72, no. 5 (August 2019): 791–800. https://pubmed.ncbi.nlm.nih.gov/31402709/.

76. Xin Wu, et al., "Allium Vegetables Are Associated with Reduced Risk of Colorectal Cancer: A Hospital-Based Matched Case-Control Study in China," *Asia-Pacific Journal of Clinical Oncology* 15, no. 5 (October 2019): e132–2141. https://pubmed.ncbi.nlm.nih.gov/30790463/.

77. Ruth Clark and Seong-Ho Lee, "Anticancer Properties of Capsaicin Against Human Cancer," *Anticancer Research* 36, no. 3 (March 2016): 837–43. http://ar.iiarjournals.org/content/36/3/837.abstract (accessed April 2018).

78. Mark Messina, "Impact of Soy Foods on the Development of Breast Cancer and the Prognosis of Breast Cancer Patients," *Forschende Komplementärmedizin* 23, no. 2 (2016): 75–80. https://pubmed.ncbi.nlm.nih.gov/27161216/.

79. Catherine C. Applegate, et al., "Soy Consumption and the Risk of Prostate Cancer: An Updated Systematic Review and Meta-Analysis," *Nutrients* 10, no. 1 (January 2018): 40. https://www.ncbi.nlm.nih.gov/pmc/articles/PMC5793268/.

80. Xiao Ou Shu, et al., "Soy Food Intake and Breast Cancer Survival," *JAMA* 302, no. 22 (December 9, 2009): 2437–2443. https://www.ncbi.nlm.nih.gov/pmc/articles/PMC2874068/.

INDEX

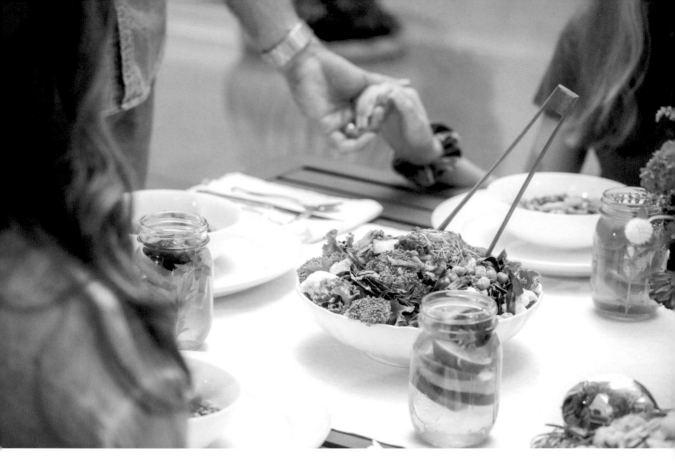

ACKNOWLEDGMENTS

Thank you to Reid Tracy, Patty Gift, Lisa Cheng, and the entire Hay House team for believing in us and our mission to bring hope, encouragement, inspiration, and a beautiful book full of delicious whole-food plant-based meals to our community of survivors and thrivers.

Thank you to the incredibly talented Justin Fox Burks for your amazing photography and creativity in the kitchen. You helped us make our dream a reality! Nailed it, bro!

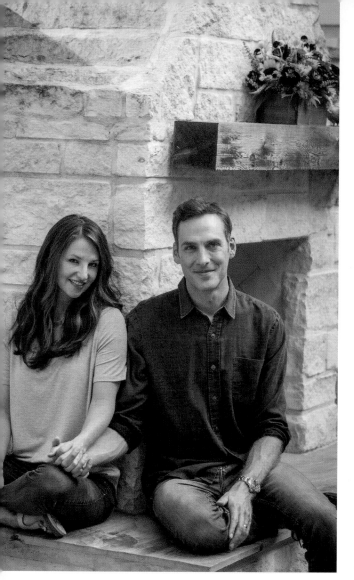

ABOUT THE AUTHORS

Chris Wark is a cancer survivor, patient advocate, and best-selling author of *Chris Beat Cancer* and *Beat Cancer Daily*. Chris was diagnosed with stage III colon cancer in 2003, at just 26 years old. After surgery, Chris made the decision to opt out of chemotherapy and chose to use nutrition and natural therapies to heal. In 2010, Chris began sharing his story of faith, courage, and determination and his message of hope that chronic diseases like cancer can be prevented and reversed with a radical transformation of diet and lifestyle. Chris is also the creator of the Square One Cancer Coaching Program, which has been shared with over one million people globally.

Chris reaches millions of people per year through his books, social media, podcast, and website ChrisBeatCancer.com. He and his wife, **Micah**, live in Memphis, Tennessee, with their two teenage daughters, Marin and Mackenzie, an 85-pound hound dog named Gus, and a tuxedo cat named Cash.

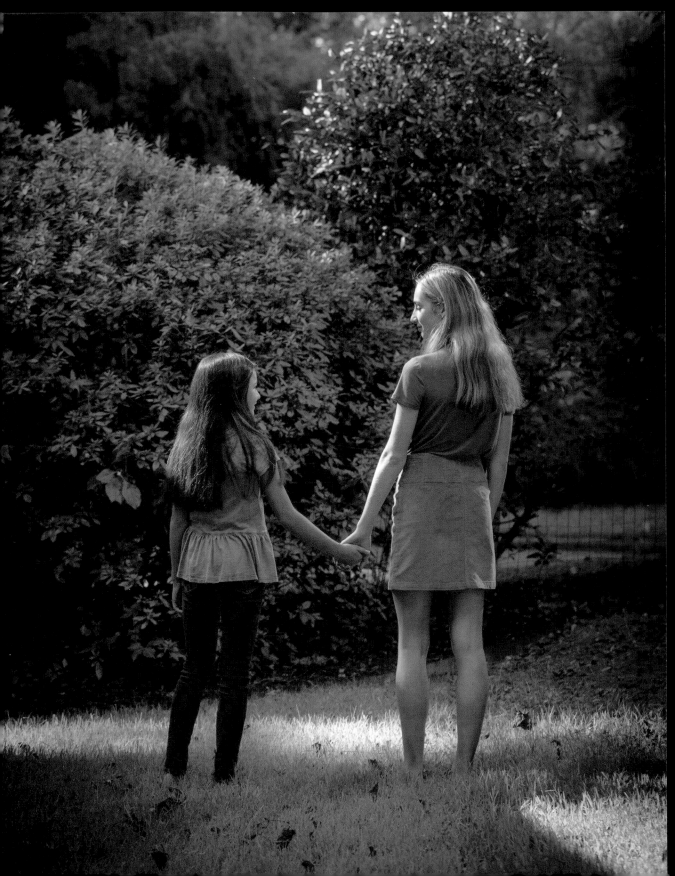

Hay House Titles of Related Interest

YOU CAN HEAL YOUR LIFE, the movie, starring Louise Hay & Friends
(available as an online streaming video)
www.hayhouse.com/louise-movie

THE SHIFT, the movie,
starring Dr. Wayne W. Dyer
(available as an online streaming video)
www.hayhouse.com/the-shift-movie

***

*CANCER-FREE WITH FOOD: A Step-by-Step Plan with 100+
Recipes to Fight Disease, Nourish Your Body & Restore Your Health*,
by Liana Werner Grey

*CRAZY SEXY JUICE: 100+ Simple Juice, Smoothie &
Nut Milk Recipes to Supercharge Your Health*, by Kris Carr

All of the above are available at your local bookstore,
or may be ordered by contacting Hay House (see next page).

***

We hope you enjoyed this Hay House book. If you'd like to receive our online catalog featuring additional information on Hay House books and products, or if you'd like to find out more about the Hay Foundation, please contact:

Hay House, Inc., P.O. Box 5100, Carlsbad, CA 92018-5100
(760) 431-7695 or (800) 654-5126
(760) 431-6948 (fax) or (800) 650-5115 (fax)
www.hayhouse.com® • www.hayfoundation.org

———

Published in Australia by: Hay House Australia Pty. Ltd.,
18/36 Ralph St., Alexandria NSW 2015
Phone: 612-9669-4299 • *Fax:* 612-9669-4144
www.hayhouse.com.au

Published in the United Kingdom by: Hay House UK, Ltd.,
The Sixth Floor, Watson House, 54 Baker Street, London W1U 7BU
Phone: +44 (0)20 3927 7290 • *Fax:* +44 (0)20 3927 7291
www.hayhouse.co.uk

Published in India by: Hay House Publishers India,
Muskaan Complex, Plot No. 3, B-2, Vasant Kunj, New Delhi 110 070
Phone: 91-11-4176-1620 • *Fax:* 91-11-4176-1630
www.hayhouse.co.in

———

Access New Knowledge.
Anytime. Anywhere.

Learn and evolve at your own pace
with the world's leading experts.

www.hayhouseU.com

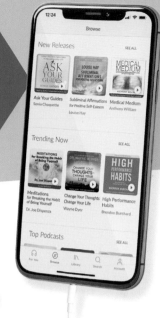